Forward

This story is for adult reading only and is for entertainment purposes.

There are many reasons a woman in her fifties has never married. This story focusses on just one of those reasons. This story is told to encourage young women who have been abused to seek the proper counseling at the earliest age possible to have the best opportunity at a normal life.

This story is also told to those that would date this type person. It needs to be understood if she boots you from her life in a moment's notice without discussion, it may just be because she was abused. Don't take it personal. Please show as much compassion as you can if you are aware of the circumstances. Because she thinks she is tough, she doesn't realize what she is doing. She thinks her abuse has nothing to do with her life decisions but she is mistaken. Trauma creates scars. Healing must be sought in proportion to the size of the scar.

If the proper therapy is never sought, the effects of the abuse will show its ugly face from time to time. She blames all men for what one did to her. The fact is, her attacker is still controlling her. Even after forty years. The stress of these events may lead to an inability to make reasonable or rational decisions concerning men. These decisions may actually be to the detriment of the victim. Stress can be hard not only on the mind but the body's organs if left untreated.

The real Becky was offered an opportunity to influence and add facts to the missing years in this story. She tried to stop the publication of the book via attorney. It took five minutes to straighten that out, but she refused to add any facts. Parts of the book are manufactured by the writer and every name associated with the real characters has been changed.

Wikipedia

Psychological repression, or simply **repression**, is the psychological attempt made by an individual to repel one's own desires and impulses toward pleasurable instincts by excluding the desire from one's consciousness and holding or subduing it in the unconscious. Repression plays a major role in many mental illnesses, and in the psyche of the average person.[1]

Special Thanks

Linda Hodges, MA, NCC, Licensed Professional Counselor
and
Carolyn Mitchell

Childhood

Becky was born in the fall of 1962 in a tiny town in central Kentucky. It was typical for the times. She played as a little girl would in those days. Her parents were still living on love at the time and did what they could to survive. There wasn't much to do for entertainment in those days. There was no money to do anything with anyway. Grandmother would help a bit when she could. People just spent time with their families. Becky had a sister, Kim, a year younger than her. Kim would become her best friend for the next 2 decades. Another sister, June, came along three years later. Her father still wanted a son. Every man does. He would treat Becky much like a son until she reached puberty.

Becky liked to play with dolls like all little girls do. She also liked to play and wrestle with the boys. She never turned down an opportunity to play with the little boys and their toy cars and trucks. Her daddy was raising a bit of a Tom Boy. He didn't have a son so he did the best he could with his oldest daughter. He taught Becky how to fish and enjoy the peacefulness of the water at an early age. She was close to her father in the early days even though his discipline was a bit extreme at times.

He introduced her to blackberry picking in August when she was 6 years old. Daddy liked to have a beer when he picked blackberries. (Living in a house with four women would make it easy to have a drink). She just loved spending the time with daddy. It got her out of the house. It was during this trip she learned what chiggers were. She had so many, they almost looked like she had the measles. She had already had the measles earlier that year. She had finished the first grade and already had all the childhood diseases. Of course, both of her sisters had the same diseases. In those days kids built a much better immune system by letting their body fight the diseases. A few did die but still fewer than the immunizations kill today. The immunizations don't build a healthy immune system.

In the summer they would visit friends in the nearby town. They were better off and actually had a sprinkler the kids could run through. Becky was always there to help her mother and father in the garden. She liked playing in the dirt more when it was freshly tilled and not later in the year when it had hardened from all the rain.

Her fathers' older brother lived only a few miles away. They would have frequent family picnics at a park with swings and teeter totters. Becky would play with her two older cousins Jimmy and Kenny. She looked at them as the big brothers she never had. She looked up to them. Once at a picnic, it rained some and created mud all the kids could play in. There were ass whoopins all around for the kids that day. Becky's father spanked her but not rough that day. She was his favorite, even though parents aren't allowed to have favorites. The picnics would be remembered by Becky her entire life. She would sit for an hour on hot summer evenings listening to her voice vibrate in the fan.

When the cousins would come to visit Becky's house they would kick a ball some. Jimmy and Kenny taught her to catch June bugs. Tie a thread to their leg and fly them in a circle. That was the closest thing kids had to a remote controlled aircraft in those days. Becky used to take sides with her cousins and scare her little sisters with worms, until one day, when June ate one, and all the kids got in trouble again.

In the winters Becky's mother, Stella, kept the kids busy with indoor games. Stella tried to encourage Becky to read more. It was obvious to her parents that Becky was smarter than the other kids. Becky's mother encouraged her girls to play dress up. She started teaching Becky very early to cook. She would tell Becky, you need to be able to cook to keep your man happy when you get older. Stella also encouraged the all-important naps. It wasn't just the kids that needed the rest. Stella always made sure they had a tea party once a year. Becky's fall birthday was a good time to plan this around.

Ultimately, Becky's father just couldn't make enough money to stay in the small farming community. Becky's uncle and his family moved to central Indiana the spring of 1968. There were jobs and new factories nearby. Becky's parents packed up the family four months later and followed. They settled an hour from Indianapolis.

In the new town

In grade school some girls are shy and need help asserting themselves. This was never Becky's problem. It was a small town. Everyone knew each other and only the dirtiest of secrets were ever kept. Becky remained an Honor Roll student throughout grade school. One reason she did this was to make her parents happy and to seek their approval. Making kids feel loved was lacking in a lot of homes back then. Becky's was no exception. She spent a good portion of the fourth grade doodling because school was not much of an academic challenge for her. She and a friend sat between two boys that had been put on different sides of the room for talking. The boys began communicating in sign language. Becky and her friend learned sign language in just a few days. This spoiled the boy's secret way of communicating. This was just an example of what smart and bored kids do in school. They were getting a little big for "Duck, Duck, Goose, now".

Like a lot of the young girls, Becky wanted to be liked by most of her classmates, girls and boys. She did what she could to socialize and cut down on some of the turmoil between other students.

Becky was eleven now. This was the year she got her boobs. She was a very attractive, lean, young lady. She was a bit taller than the other girls. This is also the year she got her braces. Her parents let the local dentist talk them in to letting him do the orthodontics. He pulled Becky's first upper molar on each side. He said there wasn't room for all the teeth to fit. The end result created just a bit of a shark effect. No real orthodontist would have straighten her teeth that way. Regardless, she turned out to have a beautiful smile. Her friends would always love seeing her smile. Her smile made her face glow.

Becky's mother had given birth to three girls. She did not feel she was still the sexpot she was when she got married. It was discovered that Becky's father was seeing another woman that year. After nearly 13 years of marriage. There was a lot of angry emotions at Becky's house and she really didn't like to see her mother or her sisters in this kind of pain. Becky decided, men that cheat on their wives are just a bunch of assholes (regardless of the reasons).

Becky got her period just before her twelfth birthday. She was growing into a beautiful young lady. Her father showed a bit more respect, but she was afraid of him because he would be abusive when he was drinking.

Age 12

Christmas 1974. Cousin Jimmy was home on leave from the Army. Becky turned twelve a month earlier. Jimmy's family, including his brother Kenny, came for a visit.

Difficulties at school were not discussed among family back in those days. Kenny was having difficulties at school. He was a straight C student and just didn't like school, except for the pretty girls. The kids made fun of him. Even some of the girls. He had dirty blond hair like his mother. He had a gap between his buck teeth (lots of kids called him Bugs Bunny) and he had one ear that was twice the normal size. It had some big brown freckles on it from where he had sunburn as a little kid. Before Jimmy left to go back to the Army, he gave Kenny two condoms. Jimmy told Kenny, if he ever had the chance to be with a girl, to make sure and use one of the condoms. Jimmy was trying to make his brother feel good and maybe teach him something at the same time. Jimmy didn't know Kenny was caught having sex with his 11 year old sister that year. It had been going on for 2 years. Mother and father gave him the ass whooping of his life and told him it better never happen again. Kenny was about to turn seventeen.

Near the end of March, Kenny came by driving their family car. Kenny had just gotten his driver's license. He came in and said hello to all. He asked Becky if she wanted to go for a ride around town? Her parents said fine, and the two youths took off to tour the big city of eleven hundred. Kenny went straight to the nearby park at the lake. It was almost dark and being March, it was still cold. The park was deserted. Kenny pulled the car to a deserted area. He and Becky had been talking along the way. She looked at him as a big brother. She thought it was cool to be out riding around town the way some of the bigger kids do. As soon as Kenny put the car in park, he shoved Becky down in the seat. Her head was toward the steering wheel. She said, "What are you doing"? Kenny told her to shut up and be quiet. This scared Becky and she complied. Kenny pulled her pants off. She resisted but would regret later not putting up a better struggle. Kenny put on one of the condoms his brother had given him. He got on top of Becky and very roughly penetrated her. Becky had never even used a tampon and it hurt a bunch. She was telling him to stop. He told her to shut her month again. He didn't want to hear another sound out of her. This was terrifying and would haunt Becky forever, subconsciously. Becky would be totally silent while having sex for the rest of her life. Not even one moan like most other women.

While he was pumping on her, he told her she was very pretty and he loved her. Becky was just praying to God it would stop soon. She lay there staring up at that one big ear until he started drooling on her face. She turned her face and covered it with her hands. It took Kenny about six minutes to affect this beautiful little girl's life forever. It seemed like hours to Becky.

Kenny finished, and as they were putting their clothes back on, he pointed out her parents would not approve of what she'd just done. It needed to be their secret. They both would be punished and never see each other again if she said anything. What they had done was for adults and she needed to be quiet. He told her she was a real woman now. He drove her home and let her out in front of her house. He then drove the short distance home to the next town. He was smiling the entire trip.

Becky went inside. Her mother asked her how the ride went. Being the quick thinker she was, she said it was too cold and none of the other kids around town were outside. Becky felt dirty, sick actually. She then told her mother she was going to take a long hot bath. She spent 45 minutes in the tub trying to get the dirty feeling off her. Becky hid her bloody panties and threw them in the garbage later when she knew her mother was busy. She made sure to give her father a big hug before she went to bed that night. She felt like she had betrayed him. Her nightmares were just about to begin.

Becky could not tell her parents. She didn't trust her father to handle it in a rational way. She was afraid of being brutally punished herself. She just was too embarrassed to tell her mother, and she didn't want her parents arguing over this.

Memorial Day was just two months later. Becky's family and all her cousins were at the local park. Becky did not understand the mentality of a sexual predator. After the gathering had been going on for a while, Kenny saw Becky near the edge of the woods. When no one was looking he took her by the hand and dragged her into the woods about 60 yards. Kenny had been to the park the day before and had hidden a blanket in a plastic bag. When they got to the area Kenny had chosen he told Becky to stand still and be quiet while he unfolded the blanket on the ground. He told her to take off her pants but she just stood there. Frustrated, Kenny unsnapped her pants and pulled them down. He pushed her down on the blanket. He put on a condom and mounted Becky like he had done two months earlier. Becky could not stop the tears in her eyes. Once again, she prayed to God it would be over soon. When Kenny finished, he assured her she would like it more each time they did it. Becky didn't seem very convinced. The two sneaked out of the woods and rejoined the party.

The party was over for Becky. She sat near the adults the rest of the day. She sat quiet unless spoken to. Her mother asked her what was wrong and she just told her mother she didn't feel well. Becky felt dirty and she needed a bath. The party soon ended and everyone went home. Once again, Becky took a bath and made sure to hug her father before she went to bed.

Six weeks later there was a small Fourth of July party at Becky's house. As it neared dark, Becky's parents and her aunt and uncle left the kids to visit friends for a few hours. Kenny was put in a babysitting position. There were other neighborhood kids playing in the area. Kenny forced Becky into the barn at the back of the property. He told her to not make a sound. He felt the need to repeat that a few times while he forcefully took off Becky's clothes. This time he was even rougher than before. He was out of condoms so he didn't bother with one this time. This time while he was raping her, he also bared her chest. Something he had not done before. Still, it didn't take long for Kenny to finish. As always, Becky just prayed for it to be over quickly.

This time he was rough and she was scared he was going to hurt her. Even with these fears, she made it clear as they were putting their clothes on, she was not happy with him. She had not done this before. She had never been so scared in her life. She was angrier than before. She was growing up and beginning the attitude to protect herself. This would be the start of a lifelong commitment to do just that. They returned to the neighborhood celebration. Becky had three male dolls at home. The next day she tore off their heads, one at a time, and put them in the trash. This time she had new nightmares about explaining to her parents how she, at age twelve, had gotten pregnant.

Labor Day weekend, Kenny's brother Jimmy came home from the Army to visit. Jimmy asked him if he had ever used those condoms? Kenny told him that he and Becky had been having sex all year. Kenny said, "She is hot and she loves it". He planned to do it a lot more and for a long time. Jimmy explained to him. She is your cousin. Even if she likes it, it is wrong. You need to stop. You don't have sex with your first cousin. It just ain't right. This gave Kenny a new opinion on the situation.

During the next year and a half, until Kenny left for the Army, three young girls, ages 12 and 13, went missing. All were within 18 miles of Kenny's house. All were slender. All had dark hair. Just like Becky. The police never had a suspect in these cases.

Becky never allowed herself to be alone with Kenny again. When the cousins came to visit she did not play. She stayed inside and watched the card games or whatever the adults were doing. Becky would cry when the cousins came to visit. Her mother saw her once and asked her what was wrong and why she wasn't outside with the other kids. Becky happened to be on her period. She told her mother she was cramping and didn't want to go out. Becky was afraid Kenny was going to assault her sisters. She watched when she could through the windows. She never knew if he assaulted her sisters because no one ever spoke of what happened.

That beautiful smile would forever hide a horrible secret. It would take a few years to get that glow back on her face.

Growing into an adult

Becky tried to be a normal 13 year old. The nightmares were not every night now. She continued avoiding her cousin and kept an eye on her sisters when she could. She was determined to not let this get her down. She smiled when it was appropriate, although she was hiding a great secret behind that smile. She tried just to be a kid her age. The whole time becoming what she thought was a tough, standalone type girl.

Becky was fourteen and a freshman in high school when she became a cheerleader. It was a small school with no football team but she got to cheer at basketball games and other events. She needed to smile a lot being a cheerleader so she really was able to develop a beautiful smile. That glowing smile wouldn't return for another year or so.

Some of her older friends were already starting to date. This is something that scared Becky. She never wanted to be alone with a guy again. She watched her friends and did some group activities with the cheerleaders. She was comfortable with this for now. By the time she was sixteen, all her girlfriends were dating. She was left out of some of those conversations because she had no boy to talk about. Many of her friends dated guys in their class, but many dated guys a year or two older. Some girls wanted a more experienced guy. A little more of the childish way boys act had already worn away with these guys. Becky's father had on occasion made the statement he didn't want his daughters dating. He was kidding a little but was concerned like most fathers. He didn't know his oldest daughters secret. He would go to his grave without that knowledge.

Becky's mom threw her a 16th birthday party. Becky's mother had a talk with her on who to invite. She told Becky to make sure and invite a boy for every girl she invited. She told Becky it would just make for a better party. She also looked Becky in the eye and told her, don't listen to your father. It's okay if you start dating.

Becky was scared to death of ever not being in control around a man again. There was a neighborhood kid she had been watching and talking to some. He was a year and a half younger than Becky. He was actually a little shorter than Becky at this time. He had the long hair which was typical for the day except for those who had strict parents. He was trying to look like John Fogerty. He was small in stature, just a tad overweight, and wore glasses (a sign of weakness to some). Becky was thin. Thin was more typical in the 70's than it is today in high school. Becky would remain skinny until she went on the pill a year later. He was not a loud kid but tried to be witty when he could around Becky. Becky felt least threatened by him than all the other boys. Her friends were dating the big strong boys but Becky decided to make sure she invited Harry (the neighborhood kid) to her party.

The party went fine. It signified to all (including her father) Becky was growing up. Becky started spending more time around the neighborhood with Harry. She was feeling more and more like he was harmless. The next spring they started kissing and a month later she started letting Harry touch her some. Not too much for a while but she enjoyed what they were doing. She didn't want the nightmares of getting pregnant to come back. She began practicing oral on her young man to make him happy and to keep him from wondering to any other girls. All the other girls were doing it, and more. This went on all summer. Becky decided she was going to have sex for her seventeenth birthday. She sneaked off to the city a couple of weeks before her birthday to see a gynecologist. She wanted to go on the birth control pill. The doctor had no problem with this but explained she needed to be on the pill a full month before it actually would work for her. She was a bit disappointed but the birthday sex would just have to wait a few weeks.

Becky had saved enough to buy a car that seemed to run regardless of what it sounded like. Her parents paid the insurance. She was able to get a job at the local skating rink where she worked as a guard for two years. (This also put her in the middle of all what is happening in the small town. This may have contributed also to her being the Home Coming Queen her senior year). She could drive her and Harry out on dates now. Harry asked her to go to the park (where she had first been raped) but she told him she really didn't like that park. There were plenty of other places.

Harry had hinted once if she had been with any other boys or if he was the first? She just said, you are my first boyfriend. After over a full month on the pill, Becky took her man to a secluded spot to park the car. She made it clear, it was time. They sneaked around like this, and once in a while having moments alone at home where they could be young and sexual. They learned at a local lake the summer after she graduated that water was not a good lubricant. They were kids and did everything other kids do. Just before Becky graduated high school, one day immediately after they had sex, she told Harry she had been raped by a relative. It seemed she would sometimes think of the rape when she was having sex. She didn't want to say his name but there would only be a couple of main suspects for Harry to choose from.

This devastated Harry for a while. He thought he was the first. He had been robbed of that just like Becky had been robbed of the choice who to be with her first time. This passed for Harry, over time. Becky was really a special girl. He wasn't bright enough to see the entirety of her attributes. He loved her and he told her so when he thought it was appropriate. Becky never told him she loved him. He assumed from the way she acted and the great sex that she loved him. What he didn't know, and would never understand, when she told him she was raped, she wanted his support. She would never say it or understand herself what she wanted from him, but she needed him to do something to help her. He never understood this, so he would be her first boyfriend to let her down.

Harry didn't really have a plan for life like many kids growing up in the little town. This was a concern to Becky. She needed to be successful, and to do that meant leaving small town USA.

When she graduated she decided to go to the technical school in the next town. Computers were rapidly growing at the time so that is the field she dove into. She would devote her life to that. She would grow to learn it was easier to depend on a career than it was a man. Deep down she blamed every man for what one sick individual had done to her. It took her fifteen months to finish the technical school. She had a certificate and began looking for a job. She found one in the nearest city but knew she needed more to move up the ladder. Harry had finished high school by now and was asking her to marry him. She just kept putting off the answer to that question. When she was twenty-one she was finally able to get a job in Louisville. She told Harry she could not marry him and she left town.

She chose a good neighborhood to move to. It had to be affordable. She was gaining valuable experience at her job. The large apartment complex housed all kinds of people. She met a male friend at work and they were discussing getting a place together to share expenses. About this time a man was found murdered just a few doors down from her. She really encouraged her new friend Pat to get a place together. So they made plans to be roommates.

Move in with Pat

It was June 1984. Lance was asked by one of his firefighter buddies to help him and a new roommate move into an apartment. Lance was a friend to as many as he could be. If a fellow firefighter needed help, you did what you could. The moves weren't far apart.

Turns out Pats' new roommate was an extremely cute dark haired girl. She had only lived in the area for a year. She was 22 years old and Lance was 26. Lance was just being friendly. He chatted to the girl for the few hours it took to move everything. He hadn't been thinking she would be great to date. Lance was in a miserable marriage to his high school sweetheart. At the end of the day, Becky gave Lance and the other helper a hug for helping move her. That hug would torment Lance until the day he died. There was a warmth from this little girl he had barely known for three hours that he would never want to live without. A couple of weeks later Lance asked Becky out on a date. She politely explained she did not date married men. That was understandable, and Lance didn't press the issue much until his divorce was finalized sixteen months later. She would not even date him after he separated from his wife.

It was difficult for Lance to be patient. He sent her roses to the apartment for her birthday, five months after they met. That is when he learned how to spell her last name. She thanked him and he got a nice hug.

Lance had been spending as much time with Pat as Pat would allow. Anything to get a chance to see Becky. Late September 1984 Pat, Lance, Becky and a friend of Becky's, Katrina were going camping. Pat had a last minute problem and agreed to travel the two hours by himself later.

Becky, Lance and Katrina set out for the woods in Becky's little Ford Ranger. It was comfortable for the three for the drive to the Red River Gorge. They went to the spot where they agreed to meet Pat and made camp. They had a few beers around camp and settled into Lance's tent for the night. Lance slept in the middle. Becky at one point did something to draw Lance's attention. They were all kidding around. Lance was nearly up on her wrestling and had her hands pinned down. Katrina turned on a light. Lance was in his blue briefs. Katrina got a good look before Lance said, "Turn that light out". They all settled down and went to sleep for the night.

The sun rose the next morning. Pat had never shown up as he had promised. The three amigos had breakfast and hiked off into the woods. This was an area Lance had visited many times. It was a great area to use his repelling gear he was carrying. A mile away when they arrived at the chosen site, Katrina made it clear she was not getting anywhere near the edge of the cliff. She was near panicked by the cliff.

Becky made it clear she was afraid of heights, but wanted to try repelling. Lance gave her the brief necessary lesson to be safe and successful. Lance even tied her gear to himself assuring her she could not fall. The cliff was about a sixty foot drop. Lance spent 25 minutes trying to talk Becky over the edge. She was as nervous as he had ever seen a person. She never said she was going to quit, even though her progress was almost non-existent for some time. She didn't understand at this time that Lance loved her and would have taken hours if that was what she wanted. Finally, her hands and knees shaking, she went over the edge. They descended slowly together. (Hours later, Lance thought this would have been a great time for a first kiss. Hanging 40 feet above the ground. Would she really have told him no)? They reached the ground safely. She had a great smile and hugged him thanking him for making her go through with it. He said, "I didn't make you. You wanted to do it". She insisted on doing it two more times before they stopped. She was much faster and more at ease after the first time.

They explored the woods that day and returned to camp. A few more beers were consumed and all were pals at camp.

The next day they packed up camp and drove to another part of the forest to view the scenery. The leaves were just starting to change. It had been a great weekend for the three.

Dating Lance

Lance's divorce took ten months to make it through the courts. He needed to bring a witness to the court to prove who he was. Lance asked Pat, Becky's roommate. He wanted to avoid any question from Becky that his divorce was final.

Halloween was only a week away. Lance and Becky went out for their first date. They went to a steak house for dinner. After dinner they went to a party of locals that Lance was friends with. There was beer. Becky was the only girl Lance had dated that liked beer. They began holding hands during the night and Lance was seen out for the first time as a single man. He had married his high school sweetheart. Few of those relations last forever, like many of us plan for them to last.

After some time at the party Lance and Becky strolled out near the car, alone. They began to get close. Some hugging and such. Close to each other's faces. Becky brushed her lips across Lance's. Was she teasing Lance or teasing herself. She did this a few times before settling in on Lance's lips. The two kissed for a couple of minutes. Turns out they were both pretty good kissers. Lance suggested they get in the car. They got in his car and kissed solidly another 30 minutes before Lance began to rub the inside of Becky's thigh. She let him rub her crotch just a few seconds then she stopped him. She said, "Not tonight okay". She said, "You come to my place tomorrow night at 7". Lance was cool with that. They kissed another 20 minutes before Lance drove her home and got a big hug and kiss goodnight.

Lance arrived back at Becky's before 7 the next night. He didn't take any protection. Becky had left her birth control pills on the kitchen table a few times where Lance could view them. They kissed at the door after she locked it behind him. She was dressed very relaxed looking. She had on a long loose tea shirt with no bra and some loose "easy to fuck me" fitting shorts. She took him by the hand and almost dragged him to the bedroom. Turns out she had enjoyed Lance being around all those previous months. She was about to let him know it.

They went straight to her bed and kissed for 20 minutes before the rubbing started. Lance wanted to pull those shorts off and go down on her, but she resisted some with the pants coming off. That would have defeated the purpose of wearing those particular shorts. Lance was about to explode. He had been waiting 16 months for this. He rolled over on top of her and she gave no resistance. He easily found his way through the crotch of the shorts (with no panties) and began giving her all 8 inches. Their lips lined up well after Lance had penetrated her. Much better than the shorter women he had dated. Lance was only able to last about 12 minutes this first time. It was a passion that Lance could never forget. When he rolled off her to catch his breath, Becky sat up in bed and said, "When I was twelve, I was raped by a relative. Three times. I had to tell somebody. I am not going to tell you his name in case you ever come to my hometown. I used to cry when they came over". Lance was a bit blown away with the information. He began wondering, how does she separate that from what he had just done to her?

Becky reached over and pulled a beer from the bedside cooler. Lance was impressed. A little red-neck romance. She had beer and her own bathroom. There was no reason to leave the bedroom. They chatted but she offered no other details and Lance wasn't about to ask. Lance didn't understand at the time that she was asking for his support. She may even have been asking for him to help expose what had happened to her, but that wouldn't become a of belief of his, until years down the road. Lance began kissing her again and kissed his way down far enough that she let those shorts come off this time. He went down on her. He stayed a little high because he had just been down there and he didn't stay long enough to finish the job. This was the only time, ever, that he didn't take her to orgasm when he was down on her.

He inched his was back up on top of her and penetrated her again. He lasted nearly an hour this time. After he finished they lay cuddling and talking for another 45 minutes. One of the things he told her was he needed to find out how to turn her on. He really enjoyed being with her. She looked him in the eye and said, "You know how to turn me on. Don't worry about that." It was starting to get late and Becky needed to work the next day. They kissed all the way to the front door and said their good byes. Lance didn't know it at the time but she would be the love of his life. Becky didn't have any long term plans. She had a few one night stands since she moved to the big city, but Harry had been her only real relation before Lance.

Becky and Lance dated every week. It quickly grew into a serious relationship. Becky took Lance to meet her friends at parties. Lance took Becky to meet friends and family at parties. Becky never took Lance to her hometown to meet her family.

They cooked dinner together. They went roller skating. Becky had been a guard at her hometown skating rink for two years. Lance still fell down a bit when he tried to do anything other than just skate around. They went some places with Pat and his girlfriend. They did a charity event for kids with Katrina near Christmas. They went to a couple of movies. Becky didn't seem to be a big fan of the movies. They laughed and cut up almost constantly wherever they were together. People thought they made a great couple.

They danced at a local club that played 50's and 60's music. Lots of twisting and energy exerted on the dance floor. They even did a little dirty dancing. This was the year before the movie hit the screens. If it was a slow song, it was common for Becky to rest her head on Lance's chest as they danced. She found comfort there. Lance was over six foot two and was working on his black belt. He had a 36 inch waist and 48 inch chest. Two-hundred and twenty-seven pounds of lean muscle. He had made it clear he loved her. Where could she feel safer? Becky seemed to love Lance, although she never used the words. She had trusted him to know her secret. A secret she did not want her hometown or her parents to know.

Becky had some friends that were going to a Valentines dance. She asked Lance to go with her. This was the first time the two really dressed up to go somewhere together. Becky was impressed with Lance in a suit and she made comment to that effect. Becky was dressed to kill. She had on bright red lip stick and Lance was looking forward to her needing to apply more. They had a nice steak dinner that evening before they went off to the dance. They danced nearly every dance. They took their breaks when the band did. The band was playing their type music. Mostly 50' and 60's music. After the dance they went back to Lance's place.

Lance had a king size water bed. They kissed and played around for a while before Lance went down on her. Even though she had been dancing and sweating, she never had any odor like many women would have. After she had her orgasm Lance rolled over to rest a second. Becky rolled on top of him. She kept grinding on him all the way to the end. Lance was a little tired from all the dancing. It took him about 50 minutes to orgasm. When Becky came back from the bathroom she told Lance she was bleeding. Lance was the only person she had been with that could hit bottom on her. Lance apologized and asked if she would be okay. With concern, she said yes. (In his mind, Lance was on the bottom and wasn't fully at fault for causing a tare in her. Becky had been more aggressive this night than usual).

Becky asked Lance if he wanted to go to a Hank Williams Junior concert. Lance was excited. He hadn't gone to many concerts. He bought the tickets and Becky paid for dinner before they went off to the concert. In the parking lot before the concert, Becky talked Lance into smoking a marijuana cigarette. Lance had done this a couple of times in private and had trouble even sitting in a chair afterwards. Lance was with Becky and would do anything with her. They sat in her little truck and smoked the joint. This was Lance's first (and only) smoke in public. Lance was so overtaken by the marijuana he had to let Becky lead him into the building. He took Becky by the elbow and followed her in. As they approached security the chief of security yelled to all his workers (pointing), "Those two are stoned. They won't be any trouble. Just let them on through". They made it through security and Becky lead Lance to their seats. It wasn't quite the nose bleed section but it was certainly a nice elevated view. They sat and enjoyed the great concert and 22 bags of popcorn.

One night Becky and Lance were in her bedroom. Pat and Pam were in his room. All that separated them was a couple of sheets of drywall. Not much to kill the sound. When Lance had his orgasm he made a bit of a sound one makes occasionally when finishing great sex. Nearly an hour later Lance and Becky joined Pat and Pam in the living room. It took an hour because Lance and Becky liked to cuddle after sex. Becky sat down first then Lance. Pat asked Lance if he was okay? Lance said, "Yes, why?" Pat said, "A little while ago it sounded like you were in a lot of pain." In less than a split second (it was obvious she had this on her mind already) Becky said, "I'm gonna stick a sock in his mouth." These were the fun times they so frequently enjoyed together.

Lance and Becky would learn a few things from each other during their relationship. Lance had taught her how to repel down a rope and tried to teach her he would always be there for her if she needed him. Most every time Lance and Becky crawled into bed for sex, Lance went down on her. He loved doing that. She got tears in her eyes when she had an orgasm. When the lights were up, Lance enjoyed looking at those tears. When the lights were off, he often would run his thumb to the corner of her eye to feel the tears. He always enjoyed giving her pleasure even more than what she did to him. Lance suggested at the start of sex one day that she sit on his face. She kept crawling up on her hands and knees not giving Lance the angle he needed. Lance finally took her hands and told her to put her hands on the headboard. He told her to face the wall honey. It's like riding a horse. Once she got into position she quickly realized she enjoyed riding horses. It was obvious to Lance no man had ever trusted her to do this before.

Pat and Lance's birthdays were 2 days apart. They had a birthday party together the previous year before Lance and Becky were dating. They were planning another. Becky had borrowed a cute brown skirt from her buddy Katrina upstairs.

After she dressed, Becky asked Lance how it looked. Lance learned the correct answer is always, "its beautiful honey". The correct answer is not, "it makes your ass look three sizes bigger than it really is". Becky, with one hand, grabbed the skirt and ripped it off. She needed to find something else to wear now because Lance was still learning how to be that perfect guy. They went to the party and had the ball they expected to have.

The next night they were back at Pat and Becky's. They hated to take that third beer keg back still half full. There were four of them trying to drink as much of the beer as possible. It turns out there is a lot of beer in one of those kegs. A lot of beer. They were not able to empty the keg.

The week after Thanksgiving, Lance and Becky spent Tuesday and Wednesday evening together as they had many nights the previous year. Becky had gone home to her parents' for Thanksgiving, as expected, and Lance had no reason to be suspicious of anything. Becky had been contacted by her old boyfriend, Harry, and invited him to her place the next weekend.

Before Lance left that Wednesday, after a great dinner and fantastic sex together, Becky asked him not to come over the coming weekend. She would be "busy". He said, "No problem," although it was Lance's weekend off. He only got every third week end off from work and they always spent most of those days together. Lance would learn she used the word "busy" when she didn't want him to know what the hell she was doing. Lance spent the next day traveling to the other side of town to buy Becky a 45 recording of <u>STAND BY ME</u> by Ben E King. Becky wanted the record and Lance got it for her. He dropped it off with Pat. It was becoming common for Lance to run daytime errands for Becky. He picked up her laundry and lots of things, including "cream rinse". What the hell does a guy know about "cream rinse"? It was easy to run her errands because he worked night work.

Lance was renting a house from his first wifes' stepfather. She had needed a place to stay six weeks earlier and he had let her move in. The divorce had been final for a year, and they had not been together for that period. He reluctantly let her move into one of the spare bedrooms. This would turn out to be a big mistake. Much like the mistake of taking her back after she cheated on him when he was 20 years old. They were very rarely at the house together. She worked days. He worked nights and spent every minute he could with Becky. Lance and his ex-wife Lisa were at the house because Becky was "busy". Lisa seduced Lance into the bedroom and he reluctantly complied. He could not remember the last time she encourage him into a bedroom. He hadn't forgotten that when they did have sex it was really good. She had the tightest pussy Lance would ever find in his life. After they had sex, Lance began to feel he had betrayed Becky. He loved Becky now, and any relation with Lisa was over and there was no way to ever rekindle that. Lance told Lisa she would need to find another place to live.

Lance got in his car and drove to Becky's. He couldn't help but notice the car in the parking lot with the Indiana license tags. A red Camaro. He knocked on the door and Pat let him in. Pat knew Becky had company but he thought they had left together. Lance's situation went from bad to worse. Becky was locked in her bedroom with her old boyfriend. Lance knocked on the door but didn't break it down. Becky told Harry she needed to go talk to Lance. She told Harry not to come out of the bedroom regardless of what he heard. Harry said, why can't I come out? Becky looked him in the eye and told him, he will kill you.

Lance retreated to the living room to chat with Pat. Seconds later Becky entered. She had big tears in her eyes. Tears Lance had never seen before. She had her "easy to fuck me" shorts on. Lance didn't need a big imagination to know what was going on in the bedroom. Becky said, I asked you to stay away this weekend.

Lance explained his ex-wife had come on to him and he had given in. He felt guilty and wanted to talk to Becky. Pat said, "You are living with your ex-wife and you expect to not have sex." Becky said, "I assumed they were."

Lance was in tears and was making no threats to anyone. Becky asked him to leave and he did not immediately comply. Pat said, "Let's go get a beer man." As Lance was turning toward the door, Becky took a fighting stance toward Lance. Lance was hurt, but couldn't help but chuckle a bit that she thought for even a second she had a chance against him if he lost it and decided to go for broke. Lance had feet like lightning and he was extremely accurate. Lance and Pat left to get a beer. Someone else was exiting the main door in front of them. Lance tried to punch the door before it shut all the way and latched. He was a split second slow. Pat agreed to go to the hospital with him to get his hand x-rayed. Pat went back inside and told Becky he was taking Lance to the hospital. Lance realized now the Stand by Me record was for her and Harry.

Becky and Harry left and rented a cheap motel to finish what they were doing. Harry told Becky he didn't like her seeing a man more macho than himself. Becky thought, you think I am going to date a bunch of candy asses the rest of my life. This was Harry's "Goodbye Fuck" from Becky. After a night in bed with Harry, Becky took Harry to Fort Knox. Harry was a deserter from the Army. If Lance had known at the time that MP's would respond quickly to collect a deserter, he would not have hit the door but would have been on the phone to Fort Knox MPs.

Lance and Pat returned later. Pat said, "They are gone. You can just crash on the couch." About nine the next morning Becky returned. Lance woke up on the couch. She told Lance she would call him the next night. She was sorry and she really wanted to talk but she needed to be alone at this time. Lance said, "Fine." He grabbed her hand as she started to turn and told her he loved her. She just shook her head yes and headed to the bedroom.

Becky called Lance the next night and asked him to come over. When he arrived she encouraged him to go to their local dance pub. It was Tuesday night and the place was near empty. They chatted. Lance told her he wasn't surprised she had been with her old boyfriend. He had always expected and feared it to happen. He didn't like it, but it was a part of her past she hadn't finished with. She explained she wanted the relation they had for a year to continue. She was sorry he had been caused any pain by her being with Harry. She told him the relation with Harry was over. He was now possibly in a military jail, and she could never even a bit consider having a future with what really was a loser. She hated to say that about her high school sweetheart. Lance told her he was okay with it. He just wanted her in his life. They hugged and danced a couple of slow dances. They got a bite to eat on the way back to Becky's. Things got back to normal later that week. The two seemed very happy together.

They were in the bedroom two weeks later. They had taken off their clothes. Becky put herself in position and went down on Lance. She had not done this the entire time they had been dating. Lance had never requested this because he treated her with Kidd gloves, because of her history of abuse. Two seconds after she started sucking him, Lance concluded she was not new at this. She showed a deal of expertise here. The hand mouth coordination was very impressive. Near the end she started to stop and Lance asked her to finish. She continued for a bit and got just a little cum in her mouth before she stopped. It didn't seem to please her a lot. She climbed up on Lance and finished the task vaginally.

They went out one Friday night dancing. They had a lot of fun as usual. They did not have sex that night. (After the first time of having intercourse, Becky never once in their relationship told Lance "no" when it came to sex. She would sometimes tell him she was on her period but half the time, they would go ahead with the sex regardless of her being on her period). Becky was finishing up a heavy flow with her period.

The next morning they showered together. Lance watched her wash herself. When they got out of the shower, she put a tampon in. Lance pulled her down on the bed kissing her before she dressed. He went down on her. The string didn't bother him and he knew she was clean. He had just watched her wash herself. He raised her right leg and let it rest on top of him (laying almost perpendicular to her) while he licked and sucked her. He had his left hand out where he could gently rub the inside of her thigh. More importantly, he placed his hand on her belly so he could feel her muscles contracting. She made no sounds but he could judge where she was by her breathing and the tension in her belly muscles. She would get close and he would slow down. He wanted it to be slow and tortuous. He did this several times. Finally after an hour he figured she'd had enough. He finished her off. He could tell it was powerful for her. He got some tissues from next to the bed. He pulled out the tampon and mounted her the way she so enjoyed him to. When he was done and going to the bathroom, he turned, looking at her face. This was one of a few times Lance saw a look of content on her face he had never seen on any other face. Lance loved Becky and that made him happy for her to feel this way.

Sometime in mid-December Lance had seen Becky's social security number. Lance had a habit of showing off how quickly he could remember long numbers. He repeated the number to Becky. He said, "It's easier to find someone if you have their social security number."

Becky had been making plans to go back to school. She had a technical degree and knew if she was to continue to rise in her profession, she would need a four year degree. She thought Lance might be in the way of her going to school. She was letting the social security comment cook in her head. She needed just one little excuse to get rid of Lance (as if this whole time he was just a boy toy) and this was what she was planning on using. It was also a subconscious thing that she wanted his support for her abuse, and he had done nothing. His time was nearing its end. She also was growing concerned he was going to ask her to marry him. She didn't want to tell him no so she created a deceitful plan in her mind.

The group was planning a New Year's Eve party ending 1986. Pat and Pam were going. Katrina and her X were going along with Becky and Lance. Lance was always the designated driver. The six would rent a hotel just over a mile from where the party was scheduled. Arrangements were made.

Lance and Becky went to the hotel at 11 am to handle the check-in for their room. They put their luggage in the room. They started kissing. It was their first time in a hotel. Lance went down on her (he always finished the job) and they had sex. Becky had a hair appointment so they had to move along.

Becky got her hair done. They met back up for the 30 minute drive to the hotel. They were both all cleaned up. They brought their clothes to dress at the hotel for the party. They hadn't been there long and Lance started kissing Becky all over. She said, "Okay but don't mess up my hair." He went down on her and they had great sex as usual. They had a beer in the room while they began to dress.

The six went to the party and had all the fun one would expect to have at a great New Year's party. They all brought in 1987 together as one big happy group. Lance was telling jokes on the 5 minute drive to the hotel and had everyone in the car laughing. Becky had a beautiful smile and a laugh that everyone loved to hear.

When they returned to the hotel the clothes came off and bedtime began. Lance and Becky had sex two more times before saying good night.

When they woke in the morning, they had sex. They went for breakfast and returned to the room to prepare for check out. Lance started getting frisky. Becky looked at him and said, "AGAIN?" Lance said yes. They did it doggy style this time. They had only done it this way a few times before. They had sex 6 times in a 22 hour period. They were young like rabbits.

Two days later when Lance came to visit. Becky sat him down at the table and simply told him she didn't want to see him anymore. (He had just had his "Goodbye Fuck"). This was a great shock to Lance. She would never give him a reason. Lance could only assume they were just getting too close. She was getting cold feet. They hadn't even discussed marriage, although it was on Lance's mind. He had asked her once if she wanted kids and a family. She very easily had told him yes, of course she did. She wanted everything all her girlfriends wanted.

Lance didn't just get up and walk away like Becky had wanted. He continued to call some and even visit Pat a little. She had trusted him enough, their first night in bed together, to tell him her deepest secret. Now she would not even tell him, in her mind, she had turned him into her new villain. (She would have new villains throughout her life, but always covered for the one true villain in her life). She needed to get back to school and was afraid he would interfere. She could not take the emotional risk of being trapped in a loving relationship. It never crossed her mind he might actually be the type that could support her through school. Not financially. Lance was a public servant. It was very possible he could help make her life easier while she went to school. They would never discover if that were possible.

The first of March, Becky asked Lance if he would meet her at a therapist office. He was willing still to appease Becky in any way. They met at the therapist. The therapist acted as a referee. Lance felt as if Becky was accustomed to this type setting. Becky had no real explanation. She just told him she was done with him. He made mention they had sex 6 times in one day, two days before she broke up. Why would she do that if she were planning such a thing? The therapist said, "He says your actions don't match your words." Becky said, "You could have had anything you wanted that night." Lance replied, "I had everything I wanted. I had you by my side." The therapist asked, she wants to know what it will take for you to leave her alone. Lance nearly in tears said, "If she wants me gone I'll leave for one of her big hugs." He looked at the therapist and told her, "You need to encourage her to settle her rape issues." He said, "I have read many wait until they are 35 (more like in their 40's and 50's) to begin this, and that is too late to have a normal life." They hugged and Lance left with a reasonable expectation she would work on her rape issues. Lance didn't understand, Becky didn't think she had any real issues with that. Was it possible Lance had not exposed her secret like she had wanted? He did not give her the support she wanted. He had let her down just like Harry before. Maybe she was dumping him trying to make him angry enough to go to the police with her story. What was really in her subconscious that was ruling her to break up with men that loved her, in a moment's notice? She had not and would not ever ask Lance not to reveal her secret. Was this another indicator she wanted him to tell?

Lance would be haunted for the rest of his life over losing his special Becky (perhaps because there was never any discussion as to why).

College to Facebook

Becky started college just after she broke it off with Lance. She did one semester at a traditional college then switched to a college that does one class a month. She focused on school and partied less than when her and Lance were together. She dropped out of the martial arts (something that would have boosted her self-confidence). There was only so much time in a day.

Becky tried scuba diving as a way to meet men. It would have been a great way to do just that. Many of these men were fairly physical and she was reminded by her attacker she needed to be careful not to get in that position where she was not in control. She never pursued any serious diving. Lance had started scuba diving the year before to meet women but it never really panned out. Not many single women were scuba diving.

Four years after Becky dumped Lance, she moved into a new home. Her first purchase. She had only been there a few days. She came home and it was obvious someone had gone through her things. A couple of items easy to pawn were missing but nothing significant. She called the police to report the crime. The police arrived. They ascertained there was no break in. If someone took her items they had used a key. Finishing up their report they asked her if she had any idea who would have done this. She gave them Lances' name. The officer (a personal friend of Lances') asked what proof she had? She said, "She had none but felt he might be out to get her. He was watching her." She said this after four years and no problems from Lance. Was she paranoid or what? The officer firmly explained that when houses are built every contractor involved gets a key to the place. She needed to change her locks before she started accusing anyone, without proof, of breaking into her home. He also explained, she better have proof in the future before she accuses a person of a crime. He told her, it could get her in big trouble.

She told the cop she would see to that the next day. Lance had never stalked Becky. The only way he could find her address was when the new phone books were published. This was before the internet. Becky had made Lance a villain in her mind and she was sticking to her story even though she was 100 percent wrong. This was her rapist still controlling her life. Maybe what she really needed to do was to take a brick to the head of her rapist, but she seems to still be protecting him. She just didn't understand what was happening to her, because she never sought the proper treatment.

Three years later she met a man she would come to know as a "momma's boy". He was a bit of a boring wimp. She never felt threatened by him physically or intellectually. He was just there to satisfy (although poorly) that occasional sexual urge, and the need for basic companionship. She used him as a bit of a crutch while she worked on school. This relationship was never spectacular but it lasted five years until he confronted her one day. He said, "We have been together for five years Becky. Are we going to plan a future together?"

Becky's focus was school and a career. She could believe more in a career than she could a man. He never satisfied her like Lance had so she knew there was plenty better out there. She said, "Are we going to plan a future together?" She pointed toward the door and said, "There's the door. Go through it and don't come back." He left without ever contacting her again.

Becky was 32 now. She had two more years of school. A friend of hers took her to a swinger's party one night...Becky hadn't had sex in six months and was getting a bit horney. Becky went along with the idea of just watching. She was a bit flabbergasted by the orgy she was witnessing. She decided to try it. Everyone was using condoms so it must be safe. She let two guys penetrate her that first night. She also had a female lick her crotch in between the two men. She enjoyed the men but was still curious of the woman. There was no emotion to deal with among these people. When it was done you just walk away. Becky appreciated that idea.

Becky returned once a month for the next year. She would lay down with as many as five men in one night. She also took some time in this year to explore if she was gay. It turns out she didn't really enjoy the women. She decided to stick with the men. She arrived back at home one night after being with the group and four men. She felt dirty. Dirtier than ever before. Dirty as when Kenny was raping her the first time. She never returned to swinging.

For the next year until she finished College she went to the local Baptist church two or three times a month to try and meet men. This never panned out for her. She didn't understand an unmarried woman at her age was beginning to stand out a bit as someone maybe to avoid, at least in the Baptist community. Her last few years of school had taken their toll. Becky was adding a few pounds because of her in activity.

Becky graduated college when she was 34. She started square dancing the following year. Still not finding a regular boyfriend. She danced for 6 years. She started dating another square dancer. After this failed, a month later, she quit square dancing. She wanted to avoid the confrontation with the man. Harry had been the only man she was able to break it off with without it seeming confrontational. She was always the one to break it off, if she dated a man more than a few times. This never occurred to her. Why was it that the men never dumped her? Realizing she was unlikely to ever let a man control her life, she had her tubes tied when she was 39 year old. That was one concern she could put aside regardless of the fact she always wanted and expected to have children.

Becky would occasionally date for a short while, but one night stands became easier and easier. She knew the young men would always be available to screw her. She could find those at the loud bars or almost anywhere. The bars were her favorite spot. She thought all the guys were there just to get laid. She would flash that beautiful smile and offer to leave with them. She never took them to her place. That would have made it personal.

Becky moved into a nicer home in a nicer neighborhood. She was spending a lot of time at home alone. She never brought her sex partners home. The quiet of living alone let her reminisce and consider if she had made the best choices in life. She would tell herself aloud she had, but she was disappointed there would never be children like she had wanted. This told her something was wrong but she could never just put her finger on the problem. The problem was she never had the proper treatment for being raped when she was twelve.

She had told the men closest to her she was raped and none knew how to help her. She had kept that secret forever from her parents. The two people that could have given her the support when she needed it most. Maybe the guilt would have stopped at an early age, and not followed her through life, occasionally rearing its ugly head in the form of a poor life decision.

After Becky finished school she devoted more time to her career. The position she had in computer support could be stressful at times and always required her to be at the top of her game. She began spending a larger portion of her time with women and less with men. She could be with a big strong man only if she knew it would be a one night stand. She could not get emotional with a big strong man. She could not relive the nightmares of her teenage years. The only reason Lance had a chance years earlier was the sixteen months he spent hanging around disguised as Pat's friend. She had enjoyed his company, and hadn't given much thought that he would fall in love with her. She failed to realize that she was easily a lovable person. This would be a fault of hers throughout her life.

When Becky was forty-nine, she looked Lance up on Facebook. (She was hoping he might still be a trusted friend). He was one of only two men she had trusted for a while in her life. She currently had no man to trust and was fairly sure she could never trust another. Deep inside, her hatred for the abuse she had suffered was growing stronger. (Not just the rapes, but the fact until he got old and sick, she feared her father. She also had a resentment she could never voice that he could have been the one to stop her abuse, if only she had trusted him enough to tell him what had happened that first time). It was a stress she could not admit to.

Becky was tough, she thought. She just couldn't see how it made her feel or how it had affected her life. She couldn't see she was turning into an empty shell. She had a lot of fun with Lance back in the day. She had missed him the years following the break up but was always too proud (and paranoid) to contact him and talk to him. Besides, he was very emotional and she wanted to avoid any guy like that. She really missed the great sex they had together. No other man seemed to put forth the effort to please her in bed like he had. Other men were just out for themselves.

Becky and Lance had ran into each other about five times over the years. Neither had the courage to even ask for a phone number. Lance still missed her but could never tell her. He felt like telling her he loved her is part of what scared her off in 1987.

Lance after Facebook

Late September 2012. Becky sent Lance a friend request on Facebook. Lance was extremely surprised. He thought she had banished him from her life forever. The last time they had ran into each other was about five years earlier at a local theme park. Lance was in the wave pool with his twelve year old daughter. Becky and Lance chatted for a couple of minutes. Like old friends would. Then they went their separate ways. Lance accepted her friend request.

They just did some idle chatting until Lance convinced her to meet at the local DQ early one morning in January 2013. They met and just caught up a little. Becky apologized for the way she handled their break up twenty-five years earlier. Lance (still assuming she split because they were just getting too close and she was afraid Lance was going to ask her to marry him) told her she didn't need to apologize. She was taking care of Becky, and he was good with that. Lance reached out and touched Becky's hand. He looked her in the eye and told her he never thought for one second of doing anything that could hurt her. I always just wanted you to be happy. She said "She knew that."

Lance felt like she was holding something back. Both were a little anxious to see each other. Becky was fifty now and never married. Lance asked, (with a smile) so what do they call you? Old maid, spinster? She added, gay. Lance asked her to repeat what she said. She said, "Gay." (She was asking for his approval and support but he just remained neutral) He said, "Well, that thought never crossed my mind." Lance and Becky had spent a lot of time in bed doing adult boy and girl things when they were together. Lance had been with bisexual women before and they seemed to be lacking in bed. Becky was lacking nothing in bed except the ability to moan. Lance could not believe Becky was gay. Lance asked her if she was gay?

She said nope. "Still prefer men. Just don't trust them." This was her way of telling him she was bisexual. Lance didn't give it much thought until months later he saw on Facebook Becky had travelled to Key West alone. It was difficult to overlook any longer. Becky was bisexual.

Becky had been a happy go lucky spirit when she and Lance were dating. He felt she was fragile because of her assaults when she was twelve but she really seemed good when they were together. Lance would find out the next two years, after their DQ meeting, that her distrust for men had eaten away at her confidence in life. As her bait to attract men began to expire with age, she realized there were times she desperately needed affection. Women are naturally more nurturing than men so that is where she turned. It just seemed easy for her. She needed the affection. She could never hold a long term relationship with a man. She was afraid she might get herself into a spot where she was not in control of her wellbeing. These were nightmares she never wanted to relive. She just could not take the chance. As she had gotten older, what happened to the beautiful little innocent twelve year old, would reach the point that adversely affected what most think of as a normal life. She denied herself a family because she could not submit to a man or cooperate with a man to that degree. She turned to women to satisfy her sexual needs. Although this would never totally satisfy her. She never felt totally comfortable with the women (sometimes even felt disgusted) but they were able to temporarily sooth her needs. This author read once, a female (who is not gay) will not be fully satisfied with her partner until she has had his penis inside her. This is where Becky was in life.

When they met at DQ, Becky was off on a brief medical leave because she had gotten into a confrontation with two men at work. Her ugly past was resurfacing and she continues to deny it had anything to do with her current circumstances.

Lance asked her if she had ever done any serious therapy on what happened to her when she was twelve? She had not, was her answer. (This was disappointing to Lance).

Lance asked for her phone number and she gladly complied. Maybe she was looking for the trust she once had for Lance. Maybe she was hoping for more support from him this time. He was young, uneducated and inexperienced on the matter previously. She was mature and reaching out to an old friend. Lance was anxious at the meeting and didn't clue in until later what she really was asking for. The gay thing threw him off and he was already on edge.

As Lance and Becky parted ways from the DQ, Lance sat in his car. All the old feelings Lance had for Becky came rushing back to him. It was overwhelming, as if he had been hit by a tornado. He sat and cried for a minute. Not a tear had been in his cold eyes for over fifteen years over anything. He had been emotionally shut down that long. Becky had awakened his spirit to enjoy life. Lance had spent the last twenty years with his nose in his work and his kids. He had done nearly nothing to make himself happy. Lance did not understand he was about to relive all the pain caused by Becky's absence, tenfold.

Lance ran into Becky a few days later at an electronics store. They were both there for computer issues. The anxiety was gone and the two chatted in a very friendly manner. It had been twenty-five years since they looked at each other with the comfort of best friends and former lovers.

The next few months, Lance just communicated briefly with Becky on Facebook. He knew she would make a great friend. Everything they ever did together was a great time for the both. His anxiety to be with her was growing. Lance realized he could not just be friends. He wanted to taste those lips again. They were amazing. He wanted her in his life and asked her to meet him for dinner. She named a spot and time, and Lance was there. They had a nice chat at dinner. Lance had come with the intention of telling her how he felt about her. He chickened out. He did manage to get out of her that she did not want to rekindle an old flame. It just wouldn't work she told him.

Lance tried a few times the next year to get her to meet but, she refused. Early November 2014 Becky text asking if he wanted to go to a concert with her. This would be the beginning of an end. He said yes. She later text him she could not get the tickets. That night Lance saw on Facebook a post of Becky's. She was at the concert with a girlfriend. Lance went off. He thought she was fucking with him. In his mind, she was a trusted friend. She had betrayed him. She had lied to him. He thought she was just trying to piss him off. He sent her a nasty letter with her birthday card the following week. Lance had made the decision to get her out of his life forever. He could not stand the unbearable pain of not having her. He wrote a nasty letter knowing she would forever be angry at him. The letter read:

I saw your post at the concert you invited me to. I see you had tickets after all. I have concluded you were fucking with me. We always had an honest relationship and this is unforgiveable. What if I hung a banner from the railroad bridge in your home town that read,' "Who Raped Becky XXXXX". Would that upset you? I ate your bloody pussy till you came. Now you fuck with me like this. I never expected this sort of thing from you.

Lance realized about the time she was reading the letter, he had fucked up royally. She was going to hate him forever, and he would still be in all the pain of not having her. He thought this may have been the most stupid thing he had done in his life.

She texted Lance a few days later asking to talk. It took six weeks to schedule that talk because of their work schedules during the holidays. Lance had reached the point he didn't care if she had lied, but he could not tolerate her fucking with him.

When they did meet she told her story. There was a small untruth but ultimately she had changed her mind. She didn't mean to upset him. It just happened.

Lance explained he could not stand Liars, Thieves, or Rapist. The world would be better off without them all. She agreed. Lance was angry and hurt yet he still trusted her, with his very life. Lance went on to explain she was one of three women that had seen him emotionally screwed up and it was a big possibility she was about to see it again. Lance spoke to her like she was a trusted therapist.

She told him she was intimidated by him is why she dumped him. That blew him away. She said, "You had my social security number and said you could follow me with that." Lance had no idea what she was talking about. He told her he never had her social security number. He began thinking, he used to show off by how he could memorize quickly a long number like a social security number. It was probably related to that. He never had her social security number. He could not believe she had been afraid of him.

Lance spoke for an hour, in tears much of the time. He told her he spent most of the year they broke up in therapy. This was his first round of therapy. He had purchased a motorcycle and started scuba diving. He had done everything he could to get over her and it just hadn't worked. He told her he still loved her. He never stopped loving her. His life had been a living hell since she left. At the height of his depression he even jumped out of an airplane.

Becky asked, "Without a parachute?"

Lance chuckled through his tears, "No, I had a parachute. I just didn't care if it opened or not. "That went on for years. I only wished every day that Becky was out there smiling and happy somewhere. That was the only way I could see you and cope with the fact I could not be with you. She seemed attentive to what he was saying. Lance unloaded his problems on her. Some were pertinent but he over did it.

They seemed to be finished. Becky said, "Don't do anything stupid," on her way out. Lance ate half his sandwich. He could not force the rest down. He went to his car. He had been in his car thirty seconds staring at the speedometer. This new car he purchased three months earlier registered 160 MPH. Lance was lost after his conversation with Becky. There was nothing else to live for.

His phone rang. It was Becky. They chatted another 15 minutes on a lighter level. Lance was still upset and included a reoccurring dream he had been bothered by. He told her he was in deep water and was going down for the second time. God spoke to him and threw him a life preserver. "He didn't throw it right to me", he said. "He threw it ten feet away. God told me, you can come to me now or you can reach for that." Before he could make up his mind he could hear his six year old daughter screaming from the shore, GRAB IT DADDY, GRAB IT. The dream always ended. Lance felt like this was God telling him your little girl (actually 17) still needs you.

Becky said, "Give me time to digest everything."

She had no intention of ever calling Lance again. He was just too emotional. Unusual compared to the men she had experienced in life. She was uncomfortable sharing her current life with him.

The next day Lance began having visions of Becky's father in the hospital. This happened six times the next twelve days. Lance had what he calls visions since he was an early teenager. It was never a secret, but he had maybe told a dozen people or so. He could not brag about one out of a hundred visions coming true. Some of the still shots in his mind involving places were 100% correct. He never told anyone about the visions involving people. They were almost always bad news. On the fifteenth day after Becky and Lance had last met, Lance had a feeling like someone punched him in the chest. There had been no vision the day before. Lance got on the computer and googled funeral homes in Becky's home town. He noticed there were more than one listed. He very quickly called the second one and asked about current funeral arrangements. Becky's father was the only one. He had passed away the day before. Lance did not get this punched in the chest feeling until family had plenty of time to make the funeral arrangements.

Lance went to the funeral. Lance's anxiety was high. He did not know if Becky would start cursing and run him out, or if she would be civil as he had hoped. Lance drove the 154 miles to her hometown. When he saw the sign, 5 miles, his heart started pounding. It did not stop pounding until Becky gave him a hug. While they were hugging Lance told her, he felt her pain. Lance had lost his brother and mother the year before.

Becky said, "I know you do." Becky thanked him for coming. They chatted for just a minute, both seemed to be at a loss for words.

Lance asked to go up front and see her parents but she said she wasn't comfortable with that. She hoped he could respect that. He said he absolutely could. He wasn't there to upset her. He said if he could comfort her at all he would stay. If not he could leave. She asked him not to stay. He asked her to walk him to the door and she did so gladly.

Lance told her some of the pain would stop after the visit to the cemetery. Just because it was over, but the rest was all an individual thing. His father had been gone eighteen years and he still missed him. He gave her half a hug and left. He had intended to tour the town, but was so distracted, just got in his car and returned home.

Lance had a vision concerning Becky's health but he never mentioned it to anyone.

Lance met a retired psychic a few months later. He explained his visions to her. She called them "discernment". A biblical thing. God was sending this information through him and he had to share it with the people involved. He would never do that.

After Becky shut Lance out he began to write her letters. Following are those letters:

Hello,

Thank you for our recent talk. I have never been more humbled in my life by the mistakes I have made. I cannot for the life of me expect anyone short of Jesus to forgive me for what I did to you out of my ignorance. I can only hope through my stumbling I was able to explain myself.

In reference to the intimidation; I had always thought you left because we were getting too close, and you just weren't ready. I may have said those things, but I assure you, you are one of the last people in the world I ever wanted to intimidate. Outside certain instances with my work, I only recall a handful of instances that I personally wanted to intimidate someone in my life. On the other hand, just last year my son told me I was intimidating and didn't realize it. He explained just my size intimidated people. When I approach people without a smile, I can be scary. Never my intention.

The intimidation thing has weighed heavily on my mind the last few days.

When I grew up the word love was never spoken in my house. I decided as a teenager if that word deserved being used, I would use it. My kids know it well. If that word ever made you uncomfortable I cannot apologize for that. My mother told me she loved me twice. It was on my wedding days each time.

As far as stalking you, I never did. My belief is it would be harder to ride by your home and not stop, than to never ride by at all. I did send a couple of items over the years in the mail. I have no idea if you ever received them. I kept such close tabs on your career, I heard you worked at one place just before they let thousands of people go. Next I know you have twenty plus years at your current employer.

I always worshipped the thought that you were somewhere smiling and laughing. I wanted you to be happy.

You stated you were just the rebound from my wife.

You may not technically have been the rebound. I told my wife January first, I wanted a divorce. It took nearly ten months to get the divorce finalized. Ten months before you would date me. I had a couple of brief encounters in that time.

You and I split in January 1987. My feelings for you faded only slightly until the day my son was born in June 1993. I realized then, things happen for a reason and this was best. I have to stick to that, to this day, because of my children. Because, I believe things happen for a reason doesn't mean I am always happiest with God's decisions.

I cannot express my gratitude for your phone call after our talk. It was a huge surprise, and the only positive moment in my night. You asked what the positives are? It is difficult to be positive constantly when you grew up in the house I grew up in. Also, twenty-five years of my life were spent with people, to many, on what was the worst day of their life. I would like to say I was callus to all that but it might not be the truth.

You said you never gave me a 100 percent. You said you felt you needed to be on guard, I think. Not sure on that one, or how we could have had so much fun together for over a year. I think you were on guard because of your assaults when you were twelve, not because of me. I certainly never did anything intentionally to threaten you. I need to confess a bit too. I always felt you were a bit fragile and I needed to be careful, especially in the bedroom. I was afraid to experiment with you which would have bonded us together more. So, I never brought any fruit or battery operated tools into the bedroom.

I just pray I get to see your smile and hear your laughter again someday.

I guess I always looked at you as strong and level headed. I realized now you have problems too, and I truly regret any additional burden I may have placed on you.

The days are getting longer. That's always a good thing.

Try and have a great year.

Lance

Hello,

Since we can't seem to communicate well with the phone, I am writing this letter in hopes you will read and understand my position.

I may seem to be rambling at times here and off my actual subject, but please stick with the reading.

I met you in the summer of 1984. I realize now, you were just a twenty-two year old kid even though you were at least as mature as me. I helped you and Pat move that day and I was so miserable with my marriage I wasn't even looking at other girls. I enjoyed your company that day, and you gave us a "thank you" hug at the end of the day. I have been hooked since that very moment. I felt a warm heart I had never in my life felt before. Now you have grown into a special mature lady. I really don't know how to behave.

You seem to have guilt about my first marriage failing. It was gone two years before I ever laid eyes on you. I was just in denial. She was my high school sweetheart. I think you had one of those. She only wanted to have sex once a month after her period because it soothed an itch she had. She told me once she didn't want to have sex because she didn't like walking around dripping. How romantic, huh? She made me feel like I was raping her if we did it more than once a month, and I could not do that. She did not make me feel loved. I should already have been a single man when you and I very first met. At the end she finally told me my dick was too big. Well why wasn't it too big before we got married? Why not five years before we got married when we first started having sex? Go figure. She cheated on me once and we split for several months. She came crawling back to me and I regret ever taking her back. So Becky, you need to rest assured, you did not cause that break up.

One thing that bothers me is, I spent thirty years training and serving the public as a firefighter and a law enforcement officer. I spent that time as one of the good guys. The good guys protect you and make you safe. One of the guys that shows up at your door when you call 911. Even though my training might make me potentially dangerous, it is only the bad guys that need fear. Outside of training, I have struck not one person since high school. I have been in scuffles subduing prisoners, and I have never struck a one of them. It goes deep and painfully in me that you would be afraid I would hurt you. You obviously don't understand how I feel about you. I didn't hit anyone when I found my girl locked in her bedroom with her old boyfriend. I cannot imagine a better time to lose ones' temper. I thought I handled that fairly well. You are the one that squared off on me that night like you were ready to attack. I also thought we talked and moved on from that, but five or six weeks later you pushed me from your life without telling me why, until recently.

I have spent endless hours trying to figure why I could never let you go, in my mind. All I can come up with is, you made me feel special and more alive in that one year than all my other years combined. I guess my love is forever. I still love my first wife too and might be tricked into helping her out if she came to me, but I really don't want to ever see her again. EVER. The most passionate memories I have in life are sitting on your couch trying to wear out each other's lips and a couple of moments in the bedroom. A passionate moment always seemed just a step away when I was with you. I don't know how you felt or even if you were thinking of me when we were in bed, but I remember a few times seeing a look of contentment on your face unlike I have ever seen anywhere else. This made me feel loved even though you were unable to ever use the word. Hell, I was like high fiving myself knowing I had done it right. I don't know if you remember any of this but I have thought of it a million times for the past twenty-eight years.

I would like to now lay the nasty letter to rest that I wrote you. I thought you were fucking with me and had lied doing so. I am not a selfish person. I have given my very life to helping strangers, and I feel you cannot raise kids being selfish. That said, the intent of the letter was selfish. I needed to get your attention. I felt I needed to set the stage to make you an eternal enemy, because I could not stand the pain of not having you. If I made you an enemy all would be better. My thought was you would leave and my pain would stop. About the time you read the letter, dumbass me realized, all it is going to do is make her hate you. You will still be without her and the pain will never end. There will never be a resolution.

I did not realized until we met at DQ how empty or cold my heart had been for fifteen years. All these emotions came rushing back. It was really overwhelming and I still can't adjust to handling them. You brought my desire to live back, and I want to say thank you, but it has been so painful. I wanted to tell you how excited I was to see you at the Mexican place, but guess I lacked to balls. I got in my car cursing myself for not saying anything. And I said something goofy and untrue as we parted that evening. I said I was wondering if those lips had gotten any sweeter. I knew they hadn't because there was just simply no room for improvement.

Apparently my love is forever.

Miss you.

Lance

Hello,

I sent you this to let you know, I have started sharing my problem with others. Becky, you made me a villain twenty-eight years ago so you could walk away. I think you know, I was never the villain. Nor am I your adversary.

I have written a letter to a love connection type person.

Dear Phil,

I have been watching your show a little more lately and have decided to put your "Love Advice" to the biggest test.

In the summer of 1984, (June I think) I helped a friend and his new roommate move into their new apartment. His roommate was a very cute and smart dark haired female. It was not love at first sight, but when she hugged me at the end of the day, to thank me, I felt as if her heart had its own little arm that reached into my heart and squeezed saying, "we could be great together". I realized a year ago I have been obsessed with this woman since that very moment. She was twenty-two. I was four years older.

I did not make my feelings known at the time. I was two years overdue to divorce a very miserable marriage. This girl and I did not begin dating until Halloween over a year after we met. It was a very intense fourteen months until she dumped me. I never knew the real reason until January 2015. It turned out to be a huge misunderstanding, and we were both just too immature to understand how to work it out.

My obsession for her faded, but not my memories. She and I do not know the same people nor do we run the same circles. Yet, we have ran into each other five times or more. I feel a higher power wants us together, in some way. Only one of these would be coincidence as far I am concerned. That would be a meeting at a lake. We both enjoy the water. Each time was very brief and courteous. No phone numbers or anything were ever exchanged.

A couple of years ago she looked me up on Facebook and I finally convinced her to meet. It was not a great romantic setting, but breakfast at the local Dairy Queen. She had coffee. I had orange juice. We chatted for a while and she gave me her number. When I got back in my car, all these old feelings came rushing back into me and I have been overwhelmed ever since. I have asked her to meet me for a dance. She refuses. She has grown into a very mature business professional. The fact that she is now in her fifties and still single should be a huge red flag for anyone.

I have discovered that she is afraid of me to some degree. That I might physically harm her. She could never be more wrong. I have never even shaken my finger at this girl. I spent over thirty years as a public servant protecting the public. She and I actually practiced the martial arts together a few time back then. We went to different schools but the style was similar. I was a bit more advanced than her and I was a very good student. I have explained to her, I have not struck anyone, outside of training, since high school. I even spent twenty-five years in law enforcement and did not strike anyone. If she could read my mind for two seconds she would realize that whenever in a room with me, regardless of the room size, (because of my years of training) she is one of the safest people in that room. She would also understand that she is as precious to me as that ring was to Gollum.

I need very much to get the things that excite me back in my life.

When the old girlfriend reappeared, I thought I could treat her like a trusted old friend. She never gave me the opportunity. It would not have worked anyhow. I realize now if I ever get a reasonable chance to taste her lips again, I will do just that. I am old enough now to understand what she and I did years ago in the bedroom was icing on the cake. The cake, and the meat and potatoes, was everything else we did together. Those are the things I long for most. Those are the reasons I get excited about spending time with her.

I never in my life felt more at peace than when I was in her arms. I still remember one night she slept on my arm the entire night and she looked so comfortable. My arm never got numb. I can only reason the head of an angel just doesn't weigh enough to cause your arm to get numb. She never even had morning breath.

The closest I ever came to stalking her was dating a friend of hers in the hope that one day she would tell me my old girl asked about me. It never happened.

I finally pressured her a little, and now she has blocked me from her life once again.

Phil, this girl is the reason my head turns faster and farther when a dark haired girl walks by. Far more than a blonde.

What do you recommend?

Phil, I never stopped loving Becky.

Respectfully,

Lance

Hello,

If we were able to meet as I had hoped, I wanted it to be brief. Because of this, I decided to put this in writing. I tend to lose focus around you for a couple of reasons. One being, every time I see you, I am scared to death it will be the last time. This started at the Mexican restaurant when we met. I wanted to tell you that night how much you excite me, but I chickened out. As I started to write, it became anything but brief.

I always felt bad about saying goodbye to you at that therapist office that day. That is what you wanted, so I complied. I also made a huge mistake in assuming then as to why you no longer wanted me in your life. I had no idea that you thought I would be stalking you the rest of our lives (I am curios what I ever did that made you think I was that sick). You just could not have been more wrong. I guess telling you I loved you and trying to treat you so special made you feel I could never let you go through life without me. We should have worked through that with the therapist at least before we parted. Now that I know the truth, it has become the biggest regret of my life. Probably was anyhow.

Four years later when I was inviting police officers to my wedding I was informed that you had accused me of breaking into your new home. I thought it was just because I had played with lock-smithing a bit. I did not know you were scared of me Becky. This was all a fabrication in your mind and had zero merit. I had no idea where you even lived at the time. I am careful not to break the law.

When we were dating, we were both trying to finalized high school relationships. Yet, through all this, you managed to make me feel loved to a degree, I have never been able to get over. Once again we have similar concerns. The concerns toward retirement, people our age have.

You date men in their thirties or forties. (Lance was not yet letting on he knew she was bi-sexual)Whatever. You know they and 95 percent of all the others are only after a piece of ass. You know how to handle that. It's not about a piece of ass to me. It's about having someone to hold, just a few minutes each day. Just a few minutes each day to make the worries and the pains go away. If only for a few minutes. What you don't know how to handle is someone like me who actually wants a piece of your heart. I think this is what scares you most about me. Becky, what good is that big heart of yours if you can't risk a little bit of it to make yourself happy? Whether with me, or someone else. I am guessing no man besides Harry or myself has ever really tried for your heart. I assure you, no man has ever been so screwed up because he could not be with you, than me. I remember many parties, or elsewhere when I would be with a date, or even my wife, and walking across the room, away from others to cry for just three seconds, because I was not with the person I loved most.

Everyone has their fears. I am not sure of yours. Are you most afraid of being assaulted again? Afraid of the shame associated with that? Scared to death of ever being that out of control again? You are a smart girl. You know by now, it is unlikely you will just go out one night and find the man who wants to spend the next twenty years with you. I know my fears. I won't say here what they are. It is not being bullied like in high school. I have prepared for that.

Becky, I fear you are self-sabotaging your relations with men because of what happened to you. It is not fair to those who care about you. Life is full of risk. Every day when you get in that car is one of the biggest risk you take on a regular basis. Love is full of risk also. People pass away and leave us like our parents. People cheat on us which is painful and sometimes unforgivable. People can bore us nearly to death just because we love them, and feel comfortable with them. We have to protect ourselves. But we have to risk it.

I know you can stand strong and tough. I also know that close by is the façade to be able to do this constantly. I see some of your vulnerabilities. I see that sometimes you are scared of your own shadow. Maybe, because you don't have the love you need to back you up. I suspect you have felt you were on your own since 1974, when you were twelve. My motivation to leave this time is entirely different than before.

If we ever are together, even once, for anything, we have nothing to be ashamed of. I have completed an honorable career and you are near the same completion. We are both in our fifties and should be able to live with whatever decisions we make that we think might make us happy, if even for a moment.

Funny how the words to most songs only become sad when I am down. Sad how a few seem to fit almost to a tee. I will take my love for you to heaven if I am never allowed to use it here on earth.

I hate talking about this next bit, but you need a little more information. You never gave me much other than curiosity to work with. I don't know the age of your molester. Whether he was two, or ten, or twenty years older. You say you don't trust men. If he was under seventeen he wasn't a man. Regardless of his age, he wasn't much of a man. My education also qualifies him to be a sexual predator, because of the repeat offense. Many of these people never quit. They go their entire life waiting for another best victim. Some even molest their own children. Few have only a single victim. Many keep a souvenir of their victims to help them relive what they have done. He may have a photograph of you he looks at when he wants to relive what he did to you. I noticed your sister still sports her maiden name. Hopefully for another reason. (She said it was part of the divorce decree). You also have nieces. Of the five basic sex offenders only one can be rehabilitated. That is the old guy that loses his wife, his job, and then assaults a kid at camp over the weekend. All of this in a very short time. The rest will forever be worthless to a civilized society.

You never told me you loved me. You did very much make me feel that way. You told me you were holding back and always on guard. Not sure what that meant nor why you did that. I can only relate it to your assault. Did he tell you he loved you? Did he ask you to tell him? I may never know. Maybe it has nothing to do with it. I bet you told Harry you loved him.

You cannot go on thinking I am your adversary. I simply am not. Life is short and I just want to enjoy the rest of it. Neither can you think that I will harm you in any way. You are just way wrong on that. That is explained in the letter to Phil.

I offered to help you off a particular medication, because eighty percent of them contain sodium fluoride. This crap makes you stupid over time and is nearly irreversible. It is also next to impossible to find out what is in the medication you take. You asked me if I found myself making mistakes. Yes. We both have higher than average IQ's. It doesn't prevent us from making mistakes. For me the social mistakes are higher. If your mistakes are at work, they are very likely mostly related to stress. Another reason to get off the medication you are on. It inhibits the neurotransmitters. It slows down the brain. I can easily see how that could affect the job you have. I had a period or two at work where I could not do shit I had done a hundred times before. Stress destroys the body. One of my problems with my IQ is I tend to state facts. The problem is, others don't take it the way I mean it. Big downfall for me. Another downside is, my brain never seems to stop. Sometimes I think it doesn't even stop when I sleep. Thinking of you is very distracting to other things I need to be doing. One of the upsides is, I see what is happening around me. Like the tears in your eyes when you orgasm. If I were a wealthy man, I would pay a million dollars to see those tears again. The only other tears I have seen from you is when I interrupted you and Harry. The medication you take provides a large disconnect from the brain to the heart. This is certainly not helping my cause at the time.

Everybody makes mistakes. You made one when you didn't discuss I was intimidating you. I say this not because you pushed me from your life but you invented the thought that a villain (me) would be after you forever. If you need a villain in your life, it is not me. I asked you at DQ if you had ever seriously worked on your problem from 1974. You said, "No". Becky, we have to exercise our demons. Therapist, punching bag, whatever it takes. I can only imagine you did not tell your parents because of the shame that you had done something so wrong. You were twelve. That is why every state has laws to protect its twelve year olds. I don't know if you ever forgave him. I cannot imagine he ever offered an apology, because he doesn't think he did anything wrong. You never forgave yourself, and it has been a ruling factor in your life. You cannot deny that. I will always be here to talk if you want.

I apologize for dumping a world of my shit on you. Some of it you needed to hear. Much of it was unflattering to myself and I feel very stupid for downing myself.

End of letter

Following is part of the conversation after the letter was read.

Lance waited outside her work in April, 2015. She had ignored him nearly three months. She started by saying, "You're pushing it." He told her he needed to speak. She gave him that time. They stood under a covered bicycle rack to get out of the wind. Lance read the letter. Some of his questions still went unanswered. He asked her if she had told Harry she loved him? She said, "That was personal." Really? She pointed out that she took a different path than others and it was her choice. Lance told her true, but it was subconsciously influenced by what happened to her when she was twelve. She said, "There are lots of women in that building that never got married."

One out of four women are raped. Lance said, "If that is the case I bet you 50 to 60 percent of those in that building, who never got married, were assaulted before they were twenty-five."

She turned and looked at the ground when she said "It's not like there haven't been some interested parties," talking about marriage. Her voice conveyed a great lack of confidence. Was she trying to convince Lance or herself? What were their names, (Harry, Lance, Steve, Amanda, Patty, Judy)?

Lance said, "You think I am dangerous. Maybe I could whoop four or five average size guys if I didn't get blindsided. Here I stand with one little lady in front of me and she is kicking my ass everywhere. And I don't know what to do about it."

She said, "I don't understand this whole thing. Why me?"

He said, "I don't understand it either. I told you of the passion I felt. I can only guess it is because we had more in common than all the other women I dated or married combined. We clicked at everything we did, like it was meant to be. Everything we did was like we had been practicing together for years. I never wanted it to end."

There was a pause. She said, "You are hard headed".

He immediately said, "See, something else we have in common."

She turned her face away and tried not to laugh. She knew he was right.

He said, "Oh that's right. Don't you crack a smile. Don't hurt that beautiful face with a smile. Hell it could be contagious. You smile then I smile. Before you know it we are laughing and cutting up just like we used to do all the time. Before long we are sharing a beer and holding hands planning the greatest vacation of our lives."

You wouldn't want to make any more fun memories. Have you had all the orgasms you want for the rest of your life? You know I can do that for you. You know I always finished the job when I started it.

She just hung her head. She had to bite her tongue a bit not to laugh and then she said, "It is not going to happen, Lance. "

He told her, "I think you are afraid there is going to be a kiss and you won't be able to stop." She shook her head no, but wasn't very convincing.

Lance asked if he could get a pic on his phone. She wasn't real happy but complied. Lance explained he only had two or three pics of her and they were in storage somewhere. She said, "You keep those pictures, I looked a lot better back then."

She was obviously a bit concerned with herself in the aging point they had reached. Lance said, "Do you think I fell in love with the container. I fell in love with the package lady." He pointed to her head and then her heart. He said, "I fell in love with that and that heart. So what if the container has weathered some. Some of the sharp corners are more rounded. I fell in love with the package. If you think I am that superficial to worry about the few pounds you have put on, you never began to pay attention to how I cared about you."

She said, "Lance, you don't know me." (She was wanting to tell him she was bisexual but she was still ashamed to tell him even though she had once trusted him enough to tell him of her being molested as a child).

He told her, "I don't know what you have been doing the last twenty-eight years. I think though, I might know you better than you think. You hinted you were not gay. That tells me you probably tried a few girls. See, I told you I pay attention to things. You told me you still preferred men. You didn't say you were always just with men or something to exclude women. I told you my love was unconditional. I don't care if you tried a few women. I don't want to know who or how many you have been with the last twenty-eight years."

Lance got up close to her face and told her, "I told you I pay attention to things. You are special to me in ways you will never understand." It was difficult for him to hold back his tears.

She said, "You need to move on with your life." They each got in their cars and drove away. Lance could barely see to drive for the tears in his eyes.

The Interview

It was about this time Lance thought it would be nice for guys to better understand what a woman like this can be like. This is not meant as a warning to run, but a warning just to be aware. Lance approached me about the possibility of writing a book on this matter. We spoke and I was concerned that in her paranoia that she might think he has recruited my assistance in targeting her for harm the rest of her life. I pointed out to Lance, she will likely think it to be some kind of revenge. I made it clear that nothing could point to her.

After a couple of lengthy interviews with Lance I decided to move forward. I explained to Lance there were some areas I would really like her to consult on. Lance told her we were writing a book and would appreciate a bit of help from her and she could actually have a lot of influence on the book. Her answer came in the form of a letter from an attorney. She has reached a point of paranoia that defies reason. The attorney apparently told her keeping her name out of the book was probably all he could do. He threatened a restraining order. I actually chuckled out loud when Lance brought me the letter. He said, "He would sue for pain and suffering."

I thought, I have three choices. I can ignore the letter. I can reply, "Fuck You". Or I can answer the letter assuring her name would not be used, which is what I chose to do. There was no reason to further feed this girls paranoia. Here is the letter:

June 2015

Dear Mr. Attorney,

I am responding on behalf of Lance and myself concerning Becky. I consider your letter pure harassment. If I receive another, I will sue both of you for pain and suffering. With that said, let's move on.

Nowhere in the manuscript will be her place of employment, or her name. She could have saved herself some trouble and contacted me instead of an attorney. Becky's response was totally predictable based on what Lance has told me. She refuses to cooperate with males because of her attacks when she was 12. It will be easy to show her pain and suffering began when she was twelve, and she blames every male in her life, except the one that assaulted her.

I am surprised she is using a male attorney. She doesn't' realize every time she shits on a man that cares about her, she fights men at work (which cost her 2 demotions in pay), she makes a life decision based on her assault (she chose a different path than that of the family she always wanted), or crawls in bed with a woman, her rapist might as well be right there at that moment raping her. He is still winning. She fights everyone but him. She needs aggressive therapy to understand she will never totally get over this. She needs to learn to be aware not to make decisions based on what one sick individual did to her 40 years ago. Becky is afraid of her own shadow because of this person, and she appears destined to live her remaining years alone. That makes me sad.

I have dated two women that told me they were raped. Neither was as screwed up as Becky has become. I haven't seen either of them for years. They both married and had kids.

My goal was to allow her to fill in the gaps I have, and to correct that which is inaccurate. This would have taken about as long as it took her to contact you. An opportunity also, to make sure I removed anything that could identify her. I was hoping to have her double check it for me. She is apparently uninterested in this so she can take her chances on what I choose to include or miss because of whatever reason.

My goal is to warn caring men like Lance, or warn the victims of rape, the path they may go down if they choose to be tuff, like Becky, and never get the proper mental health care.

You should inform your client how a law suit works. Things like the evidence becomes public record. During the discovery phase I will be able to subpoena her mental health records, and almost anything else I want. This will include depositions from her mother, sister, co-workers, and a few other relatives. She will effectively give every writer access to my story, and they can publish parts of it at their pleasure. She will have no right to remain silent when we depose her. It is a civil trial and she has no right to take the fifth. If this is how she wants me to get the information I want, then so be it.

I don't wish to go this path but she is a mental case.

If you or any of your ilk take legal action, (I couldn't buy better publicity) I will sue for violating my first amendment rights. My intentions are not to further harm Becky. I think she has been through enough.

Any further action should be from Becky herself. Another letter from you or your type may just provoke me in telling this story around her hometown, and to the Indiana State Police. They may appreciate identifying a sexual predator in the area.

Becky needs to know her rapist may have already silenced numerous witnesses. There is no reason to believe he wouldn't do the same to her if he finds out she has betrayed him, and not kept their secret.

Very sincerely,

Rick Devine

Never another response. So we started on telling her story through Lance's and my eyes.

I asked my advisor why these women deny themselves things they know will likely make them happy? She said, 'They feel damaged and unworthy in many cases."

Fearless is not living without fear, but living in spite of fear. Fear works faster from our brain than reason. Maybe this explains some of her actions. Contacting an attorney instead of making a reasonable phone call to Lance or myself was a waste of her time.

For reading purposes, I need to include an ending to this story, so we move on from here.

The Letter

Becky received an anonymous letter. The letter said, **"I better not find out this is you. I will get you and your sisters"**.

There was an add from a local paper that read:

Law Officials are seeking information concerning sexual assaults focused in the 1970's and 1980's. One sexual predator has been identified. If you have information on this matter please mail contact information to PO BOX XXX, Indianapolis Indiana 99999. If you know of any female that grew up in XXXXX County, especially XXXXX (Becky's hometown) or XXXXX, and has moved away from the area, please contact them with the information in this add. A quick response is imperative. We can offer protection.

Becky mailed her information to the address in fear of her life and that of her sisters. A detective called, and made an appointment to meet her the next week. The investigator arrived. He made it clear he was not law enforcement but worked for an elite investigative service whose client list included the federal government. Becky told him her story. All that had happened to her when she was twelve. She told him all the necessary details. She showed him the letter she received. The investigator concluded she should watch herself. Rapist tend to turn into serial killers. If she had any big and bad friends they should be invited over frequently. Maybe ask them for advice. She said, "She knew one person who might help." The detective left.

Becky sent Lance a text asking him to call. Lance was surprised but there was no hesitation on his part. She invited him over. A long term relationship began. He ascertained who the suspect was. Kenny disappeared. Maybe he left the country. No one seemed to know. Maybe he thought he was going to prison. It is said, child molesters have a hard time in prison.

Lance began taking Becky to the range. They went almost every month for the next two years. It looked like she was getting better than Lance. He also worked with her on how to use weapons at hand. Almost anything around the house can be used as a weapon.

Lance and Becky did everything together. They were both retired, and had nothing holding them back. They traveled the Caribbean. Scuba diving along the way. They spent a month in Europe. They frequently toured on the motorcycle. They really turned out to be a very happy couple.

They lived happily ever after. NOT,NOT,NOT

This was an ending Lance had hoped for in his head. In real life, Becky kept rejecting Lance. She could see he was in pain, and just didn't know how to resolve the situation. All she knew how to do was to tell him no. She could not take the emotional risk. He needed to move on without her. She continued to reject him. If she continued to ignore him, the problem would go away just like her rape problems had forty years earlier. Time and time again, she rejected his request. They never got together. Lance thought the way to be closest to her was to suicide himself on her property. It turns out he was correct. He took the very first pistol he ever owned to his right temple. The .357 magnum detached a portion of the left side of his head.

Becky was very upset to find him that way. She spent the day in the hospital.

The very next night, Lance spoke to Becky. His voice was very calming to her, despite the fact she had banned him from her life. He told her to go to the funeral and speak to his son and wife. She could not put this off. It would be her best opportunity ever.

Becky thought she was going nuts. *"Now I'm hearing voices,"* she said out loud. Lance didn't say anything else that first night.

The Funeral

Becky dresses in her best black dress. Then she prepared for the Saturday morning funeral. She drove herself to the funeral home, courageously, like she had done most of her life.

When she arrived the parking lot was near full. She entered the funeral home. Lots of people were there to support the family. She approached the closed casket. Draped in the American Flag and the Gadsden Flag draped behind the casket. There were lots of tears around the coffin. As she approached, she saw Wyatt (Lance's son) and his wife Connie. She noticed three full size photos that stuck up just behind the coffin. The one on the left was a very young one of Lance and his first wife. The middle one was a bridal photo of Connie. On the right was an old photo of Becky and Lance at a valentines dance. She was very surprised to see herself displayed like that at Lance's funeral.

She introduced herself to Connie and Wyatt. She said, "Hi, my name is Becky. I knew Lance a long time ago." Connie and Wyatt both turned to look at the picture of Becky that was above the coffin. Connie asked, "Why did Lance request your photo be displayed here with his two wives?" Becky had tears come to hers eyes (emotion she could never share with Lance). She replied, "I can only guess because he told me he never stopped loving me. He said, he had truly loved three women in his life. I was the second." She went on to tell Connie and Wyatt that she felt responsible for what had happened.

Connie asked, "Why do you feel responsible?"

He told me he still loved me. Becky said, "He wanted to date me. He repeatedly asked me to go dancing. I turned him down. I just can't get involved with a man that emotional. Too many complications for me to handle."

Connie said, "He asked you to go dancing and you turned him down, and you think that is why he killed himself? He has danced with hundreds of women over the years. Do you not know the difference in a dance and a romantic date?" Connie was growing angry. She said, "You come here and try and take credit for what he did to himself. My husband is laying here in a closed casket because the left side of his head is missing. I can't even open the casket." At this point, Wyatt stepped forward putting his hand in his mother's chest. He told his mother, "You need to be nice. Can't you see she is hurting too?"

At that second, Becky realized that she could no longer deny that she loved Lance also. She just blurted out, "I loved him too. He took his life on my front porch."

A calm came over Connie. Family did not know yet where he had taken his life. She looked back at the photos. She asked Wyatt to put Becky's in the middle and to put her own on the right. That way they would be in chronological order in which he loved each one. She turned to Becky and hugged her. They stood there hugging each other for a minute. Connie stepped back and said, "If you brought that much pleasure to his life, I am proud to meet you. Lance requested that you sit on the front row with family, because that is who he felt you were." Becky had tears flowing from her eyes, unlike any Lance had ever seen. Becky went over and sat down on the front row which was empty at the moment.

Just a minute later, Lance's first wife walked in. She had a problem holding back her tears. They hadn't spoken in years. She walked up to the closed casket and saw the photo of herself and Lance. It was taken in November of 1975. They had been dating about a year. She said, "Hello," to Connie. Connie had only met her once. She said, "Hello" to Wyatt. She saw him only once, when he was three. Connie said, "Lance wanted you to sit on the front row with family." The tears finally broke through on Lisa's face and she said, "I'd love to." She walked over and sat on the far end of the front row.

A little while later Katrina walked in. She was an old friend of Lance and Becky's. She walked up and introduced herself. She gave her condolences to Wyatt and Connie. She noticed Becky sitting on the front row. She walked over and said, "Hello." Becky stood up and gave her a big hug. They hadn't seen each other in over twenty years. They sat down on the front row together. Katrina sat between Becky and Lance's first wife. The service was about to begin. Connie sat next to Becky. Wyatt next to Connie, and Tiffany sat down. Tiffany had been down stairs the entire time. She was having trouble controlling herself since she was notified of the event. They all sat on the front row.

(Readers, please take a moment and listen to the songs as they are listed). Wyatt had requested they start with the song "One Tin Soldier" from Billy Jack. That's how he felt about his father. When the service started. Katrina and Becky held hands. Lance's first wife, who had never met Katrina, reached and held her hand. About a minute into the service Connie took Becky by the hand. Connie and Wyatt and Tiffany were already holding hands. The minister read a brief note. Lance had left a note for the minister. The minister announced he had a note from Lance. I'll reference that now. He said, "I hope everyone that was most important to me came today. They know who they are. Many of their photographs are up front with me." He said, "I was sorry to leave each of you without saying goodbye. I have one request from everyone listening. Never turn down an opportunity to laugh or dance. That is the way it had to be." The front row lead the way in tears. There were many in the audience that could not hold back. Lance's kids had played soccer and Lance had been the team medic and also a referee. Many from the school were there to support Wyatt and Tiffany. Actually, after the service started, there was not a dry eye in the audience. Closed coffin funerals are sometimes like that.

The minister went on for just a few minutes, as Lance had requested. The minister said, the note says he only had a couple of things on his bucket list. He wanted to ride the wall on a motorcycle. He also wanted to go the Grand Ole Opry (he had wanted to take Becky there since they attended the Hank Williams Jr. concert). Then the music began to play. They played Lance's five favorite songs. "He Stopped Loving Her Today," by George Jones, "Stand by Me" by Ben E. King, "Last Kiss" by Frank Wilson and the Cavaliers, "Runaway" by Del Shannon, and Finally, "Heartland by George Straight." The minister gave a brief service as Lance had requested. He ended with a quote from Lance. Lance said, " Running from a problem will not make it go away."

The JROTC, in their Dress Blues came up front and folded the Gadsden flag. They gave it to Wyatt.

The minister announced there would be a gathering at Lance's brother's home after the cemetery. All were welcome. Then the funeral director started those on the back row to come forward to pay their final respects (Don McClain's, "Miss American Pie" began playing); as they filed by the closed casket, and then by the family on the front row. They treated everyone on the front row as if they were

Lance's closest family. Some knew who his first wife was. Only a couple knew who Becky was. None knew Katrina. They filed out.

The coffin was loaded into the hearse. He was taken to the cemetery on the mountain, only about ten miles from where he had grown up. They all gathered around the grave site. The minister said, "At this point Lance had asked that everyone sing "Amazing Grace" together to conclude the services." He continued, "He loved his family. He loved life itself. Sometimes things just don't go the way that we would prefer them to." The local Marine Corp JROTC unit (Lance had joined that unit the very first day it started at his high school) folded the American flag and gave it to Connie. The entire group sang "Amazing Grace," and began to leave the cemetery.

After the Funeral

Becky returned home after the funeral. She felt guilty Lance had taken his life. She had no idea what lay in store for her.

She had heard the voice telling her to attend the funeral. She headed the voices advice (thinking she might be losing it herself) and couldn't help but think it sounded like Lance speaking to her.

After dark she was greeted with the voice again. It was Lance. He told her not to panic. He was there to keep her company for a while. He explained he was basically an energy form, and he didn't have enough energy to do anything other than to talk to her at night. He asked, "If he could just watch TV with her, and did she have any questions?" She said, "Okay on the TV and yes she had questions." She wanted to know if she was going totally crazy, or if this were really happening?

He said, "It seems to be real to me Becky. I can't explain it well. Nothing came with instructions. I am able to see and hear you at night. I am able to speak so you can hear me. That is about all I can tell you for now. I don't really understand it. Kind of like my love for you. It was very confusing, and I didn't understand why I chose not to live without you."

She sat quietly for a couple of minutes. She said, "I am sorry if I caused you to take your own life."

He said, "It was not your fault. I had loneliness issues since I was a little kid. I enjoyed playing on the farm. Much of my time was spent by myself. I thought I would grow up to be a normal suburban kid. I didn't socialize well with all the kids. I had a few friends. I was afraid to smile a lot. My teeth were crooked. I wasn't much over ten when I started trying to make other people laugh. It gave me pleasure and took away some of the loneliness. I felt like a social misfit, and making people laugh helped me fit in most places. I would have been a stand-up comedian if I were any good. I really spent most of my life lonely. See I had that high IQ and even the people that thought they were close to me didn't really understand me. When I was eleven I thought of hurting myself. Then again at 17, 19, and 20. It started again just before I met you. I was great when we were together. I guess it never really stopped after we split."

Becky said, "This was a lifelong problem and not my fault? Why did you take your life on my front porch?"

He said, "I hoped I would be able to be close to you if I died near you. I also thought if I made you hate me, you would feel less guilty for what I did to myself. You may have been able to delay what I did for a year or even 10 or twenty. I am not sure you would ever have been able to stop me. I felt it had been a destiny of mine since I was young. I am sorry I upset you. We aren't allowed to understand everything we do. Just like you don't understand the decisions you have made because of your assaults when you were twelve. You don't understand how that has influenced your decisions. I love you so much the pain of being rejected, just, well it needed to stop. Some pain cannot be tolerated forever. It needed to stop. Please understand."

She told him, "She didn't really understand. She had been depressed many times and had never seriously considered doing what he had done. It just was never an option."

He explained, "You were depressed for things that happened to you. I was depressed for things I just couldn't make happen. I always felt like a failure. I always wanted to play music. I just could never learn an instrument. You are the only one I ever dated that had an IQ within 15 points of mine. I guess I assumed you might understand. Not the first time I was wrong. We have both been fighters. I was just too tired to keep fighting."

"So let me get this straight. I am sitting here talking to the ghost of my old boyfriend?"

He said, "Yep."

She shook her head. "*I must be losing it.*"

He assured her she was listening to Lance. He just could not materialize for her.

She told him, "One day I told you, "You don't know me". I want to tell you why I said that, and part of why I continued to reject you."

Lance interrupted, "Becky, I know you are bisexual and you are ashamed of it. I know you would die if your mother found out. You didn't realize but you told me yourself. I told you I pay attention. I didn't care that you were bisexual. I just wanted to spend time with you. You made me feel whole. You made me feel at peace. I never felt that way any other time in my life and I wanted that back. Mostly, I just wanted to hold you and feel at peace again."

"Why didn't you tell me you knew I am bisexual," she said?

Lance told her, "The way you told me was very clear that you were ashamed of what you were doing. Becky, you aren't gay. You are doing gay things because you need affection. You are afraid of men.

I know your biggest scare of all was that you might not be able to control a situation with me. I know you have had the need to control your situation since you were twelve. You were afraid my abilities would just make that impossible. You were scared you could not control an emotional relationship. That's okay. You needed to be in therapy for about ten years after your assaults to overcome this. Lots of abused girls turn gay in their forties and fifties. I'm just glad you didn't become a prostitute, and, or drug user like many become."

Becky just had a surprised look on her face.

They sat watching TV for a while before Becky fell asleep on the couch. It had been a rough day on her. She had some new things to come to grip with.

End of First Day.

Lance's energy level grew each week. Soon he was at Becky's house 24/7. He never let her know he was there during the daytime. She needed to feel she had some privacy.

Lance spent a lot of time encouraging and teaching Becky how to defend herself especially when she was at home. He also explained the other places she would be most vulnerable. She welcome the education.

A year or more had passed and Becky and Lance were comfortable with what they were doing. Lance had gained enough strength he could even help do some chores at night. They spent a lot of time in front of the TV talking and with Lance's energy level now they could even dance some.

Illegal immigrants had been doing lawn work in the neighborhood. They had been casing what houses would be the easiest targets. What time people came and traveled to work. They noted a couple of females living alone. They would be planning a night to take what they could from the subdivision Becky lived in.

What most people don't understand is how vulnerable they are all the time. A single female alone simply multiplies that. The illegal immigrants by definition are already criminals. They are working in the neighborhood for nine dollars an hour. Their motive is not always honorable. After all, these are people that left their country because their own countrymen chose not to give them a job or to help them.

Lance and Becky were on the couch talking one night. They heard a noise in the garage. Becky went to investigate. Before she could get to the door that leads to the garage, Lance said, "Get your gun and phone and lock yourself in the bathroom. Put the wedge under the door and call 911. Do it now." By the time she grabbed her gun and phone, and ran to the bathroom, they were trying to break in the door. She closed the door and put the wedge under the door the way Lance had taught her.

They broke open the door from the garage. There were two illegals that had been working the neighborhood. They realized quickly Becky was locked in the bathroom. They could hear her calling 911. They kicked the door. They busted the lock but the rubber stopper at the bottomed kept the door from opening. Becky held her foot against the rubber stop. A wise decision. Both illegals had a knife in their hand. Lance took a knife from the kitchen and stuck the second one in the back of the neck. The one closest to the door didn't realized his accomplice went back outside. He died crawling in the driveway back to their stolen van.

Being the loving person she was, Becky could not pull the trigger on her gun. Lance had not trained her well enough. Lance put his hands on the gun and helped Becky pull the trigger, striking the illegal between the eyes. He went down. His soul did not ascend.

Prior to 1990, no one had ever heard the term home invasion. It is becoming a norm in our society. Becky had every bad moment in her life going through her mind. Tears flowing and crying, she was in a panic. She began saying the "Lord's Prayer." She never took her foot from the rubber stop on the door.

The police rescued Becky from the bathroom. Becky knew who her real rescuer was. It was the man she trusted for a short time in her life thirty years earlier. He had never given up on her.

When the police questioning started, it was obvious what had happened. All except the guy in the drive with the knife in the back of his neck. Becky refused to answer what she thought was the reasoning for that. She could never tell anyone that her and Lance were having an affair. She could never tell them her lover was a dead man. She was afraid he would not be allowed to stay on earth with her. Lance had used almost all his energy. He whispered in her ear, "Just sit on the couch and just tell them repeatedly, I don't remember what happened."

The police confiscated her weapon for evidence. They commended her on the job she had done. She would not be bothered with either of these two again. They told her there were two other houses hit before hers and it was probably the same guys. At one a woman was beaten near death and raped.

She went to the store the next day and purchased a backup pistol. She had a carry permit so there was no waiting period.

A police officer arrived about a month later and returned her pistol. They explained all evidence was documented, and she could have her gun back now. She valued what Lance had taught her. She knew he helped pulled that trigger with the precise aim that was needed to stop that attack.

During the first year Becky and Lance were learning a lot about what Lance's abilities were. They began kissing after a number of months. Lance's energy level was gradually growing still. Lance was able to kiss her all over and actually make her orgasm after some time was expended. This took most of his energy. They stumbled across a better answer one day as Lance joined her in the shower.

Lance was an energy. Electricity if you will. With practice they learned the shower was their friend. Lance could almost materialize in the steam and water. Lance could suck on Becky's neck for a moment to get her flowing in the right direction. When he added his electric charged hand to her clitoris, it never took her more than twenty seconds to orgasm. Lance would notice the tears in her eyes just like when they were dating before. This became the preferred method of contact at the end of the night. (It helped her sleep well. It helped too, she knew Lance was watching over her, like the world's greatest guard dog). Spending most of her prior life alone, Becky couldn't get enough. She wanted it almost every night.

She had on a few occasions asked Lance if he could penetrate her. Lance thought he might be able to, but because he felt it was wrong, so he told her he could not.

The Ending

When Becky was sixty her mother passed away. Stella was seventy-eight. Becky went to be with her sisters in her hometown and to help make the arrangements. Becky retuned after the funeral to be with Lance. She kept herself busy during the days. She still went out with the girls on the weekends. Sometimes they did lunch together. It was eating at her that she could not tell her friends what had become the love of her life was the ghost of an old boyfriend.

There was an emptiness after her mother passed. She didn't think for a few months to ask Lance if he knew where she was. He told her he only knew she was happy and reunited with her father. He told Becky, "It is peaceful there. No bills, no worries of any type. Just peace." He reminded her the closest to peace he ever felt on earth was when he was in her arms. He thanked her for wanting him with her now. He wasn't sure he could be there if she didn't want him there.

Becky started drinking heavily for a while after her mother died. Lance asked her one night to stop. She agreed. She said, "It was just making things worse."

Lance and Becky continued their night time romance for another five years. Becky didn't know it but Lance watched her listen to songs like "Whiskey Lullaby and You Left Me just when I Needed You Most." Lance encourage her to be with her girlfriends as much as she could. She had reached the age that some had died of cancer and for other reasons already.

The spring after Becky turned sixty-five, she sat at the table one evening. She had checked what time sunset was that night. She was timing when Lance would arrive. She sat at her kitchen table. Thirty minutes before sundown she began taking a full bottle of muscle relaxers. She was washing them down with alcohol.

Lance started to stop her. He then remembered what the pain was like when he decided to take his own life. When the sparkles began to run down his cheeks he had to leave the room, so Becky would not know he was there. She took the entire bottle of pills. She sat drinking alcohol until ten minutes before sundown.

She went into the living room and put on "Whiskey Lullaby" by Brad Paisley and Allison Crouse. She stretched out on the couch. She was already getting sleepy. The sun went down. She expected Lance to arrive at sundown. Lance sat down on the couch next to her and took her hand. She looked at him. She told him she could see him better than ever now. Like when he was alive.

He shook his head yes as the tears flowed down his face. She told him the complications would soon be over. The tears flowed from his eyes as he watched a single tear flow down her cheek. He told her, "He knew. He loved her." She said, "I love you too and I apologized for ever hesitating to tell you." He said, "It's all okay. Nothing else matters now. All regrets will be over soon."

She looked at him and smiled. She said, "Can you kiss me. I miss your kisses." Lance gave her a big kiss. They kissed for a few minutes. Her last real kiss with Lance was when she was twenty-four. She could hardly keep her eyes open. Becky went to sleep. Lance sat there holding her hand. Tears flowing from his face. A large stream from each eye.

Thirty minutes after sundown, Becky's pulse dropped below forty. Lance leaned over her putting his heart on top of hers. (Their hearts were together when his love for her started forty-three years earlier) It was at his instance, Lance got his wings. It seems an angel can't guide or lead a new spirit to heaven without his wings. A minute later Lance and Becky were both headed to eternity together.

The pain was all gone. They soon realized they were chosen as soul mates before they had even met forty-three years earlier. Some things are just meant to be and we can't change them.

The End

Afterthought

Before sending this story to the press I decided to ask Lance how he felt about Becky since he has gained more knowledge of Becky's mental status. (I found him packing. He has recently retired from law enforcement and has taken a security position at a Florida Theme park.)This is his reply:

When we were dating 30 years ago I thought she had it all. She was beautiful and young. She was smart and had a big heart. Still, I hesitate to believe her magic has disappeared. There will always be a place in my heart for her. But realistically, how could I ever feel comfortable enough to commit with a woman who has proven she could dump me in the blink of an eye, without any discussion why? We all suffer from confusion, but until she can get over her fear, her anger, shame, or guilt, she is going to overreact to the tiniest thing when she is going through one of her flashback periods. She is the only one who can make the decision whether or not she and I will ever see each other again. I have a life to live.

She has had a steady relationship with three men totaling, maybe, ten years of her life. We will never know, if swift justice when she was twelve would have helped her or not. I just don't see her in a long term relation of any kind. It saddens me.

He closed with, "Tennyson said, it is better to have loved and lost than to have never loved at all." He said, "I am not sure I agree with him."

Closing

If Becky had told her parents immediately of her rape, would her life have been "more normal?" We will never know. It just seems sad that being the victim shapes a persons' life the way it sometimes does.

As a parent, I think I can tell you if my 12 year old came to me and told me she had been raped, relative or not, I'll bet money he would never have touched another person with that penis.

Maybe she was afraid her father would do something like that and it would end her family, as she knew it. We will never know. Remember, she doesn't have a problem and her abuse isn't influencing her life (though, near 30 years ago, she told Lance she wanted what every girl wanted in life). So, it's not necessary for her to discuss the details with anyone.

Becky has certainly avoided most of the worries and pains associated with a family and kids. I sometimes envy her there and only there. She goes home after work each day to an empty house. Empty of love. Each night she lays down to sleep, alone.

Fifty–two and never married.